Life After Crohn's

Life After Crohn's

5 STEPS TO TOTAL WELLNESS

Patti Lisa Fleury

ISBN-13: 9781979303866
ISBN-10: 197930386X

Disclaimer

The information and opinions provided in this book are based on my own personal experience and research and is intended as advice for general well-being. The contents of this book are not intended to offer personal medical advice, diagnose health problems or for treatment purposes. It is not offered as a substitute for medical care offered by a licensed and qualified health professional. It is also not intended or implied to be a substitute for professional medical advice, diagnosis or treatment.

The author, editor and publisher accept no liability for any injury arising out of the reliance on the guidance or the opinions expressed herein.

Table of Contents

Part I — My Story ·1

Chapter 1   The Early Years · 3

Chapter 2   Ravaged · 9

Chapter 3   A Shift in Thinking · 22

Chapter 4   A New Beginning · 28

Chapter 5   You Can't Please Everyone · · · · · · · · · · · · · · · · 31

Chapter 6   Following my Passion · · · · · · · · · · · · · · · · · · · 35

Part II — 5 Steps to Total Wellness ·41

Chapter 7   Step I: Reduce Inflammation · · · · · · · · · · · · · 43

Chapter 8   Step II: Revise Your Diet · · · · · · · · · · · · · · · · 53

Chapter 9   Step III: Repair the Digestive Tract · · · · · · · · · · 69

Chapter 10 Step IV: Rebuild the Immune System · · · · · · · · 78

Chapter 11 Step V: Reprogram your Thinking· · · · · · · · · · · 87

Part III — Food For Thought ·**97**

Chapter 12 Gut Health 101· 99

Chapter 13 The Secret to Immunity · · · · · · · · · · · · · · · · · 103

Chapter 14 Buyer Beware! · 112

Chapter 15 Stress Less From the Inside Out · · · · · · · · · · · 116

Chapter 16 The Skinny on Fat · 121

Part IV — Life After Crohn's ·**127**

Chapter 17 Blessings · 129

Appendix· 133

Part I — My Story

CHAPTER 1

The Early Years

*He who takes medicine and neglects the
diet wastes the skill of his doctors*
— CHINESE PROVERB

Some of my earliest memories from childhood were of having a mouth full of canker sores. Big, painful, open lesions throughout my mouth, making chewing and eating difficult. As a small child, it never occurred to me to wonder *why* I had these sores in my mouth. They were just part of me. And, of course, none of the doctors who prescribed the cortisone cream, Kenalog, to treat my canker sores ever asked my mother what I was eating that might be prompting my body to exhibit such obvious signs of inflammation. For years I used Kenalog cream on a regular basis to manage these pesky little eruptions, and I just assumed this was a normal part of life. Even then, as young as four or five years old, my body was communicating its unhappiness. It was clearly stating "I am out of balance and inflamed. I am giving you signs and asking you to listen." Unfortunately, at the time, nobody around me understood this form of communication.

As time went on, and we all continued to ignore the signals my body was sending, my body tried harder to get my attention. As I was entering my tween years, I started to develop tonsillitis. Repeated, frequent bouts of tonsillitis. Once again, nobody stopped to ask why this little girl was getting repeated tonsil infections. The doctor just treated the symptoms with a round of antibiotics. From the age of about 11 or 12, through to 14, I would take five to six courses of antibiotics/year. Once I finished the antibiotics, my tonsils would be good for about six weeks and then they would start to get sore, inflamed, puffy, and painful all over again. The pain made swallowing and eating extremely uncomfortable. When the pain became unbearable, my mother would cart me off to the doctor and he would prescribe antibiotics — again — and I would repeat this ridiculous pattern for years and years.

As a result of the constant use of antibiotics, I started developing raging yeast infections. Any good gut bacteria I might have had at that point was wiped out, courtesy of my continued exposure to antibiotics. My digestive tract was now home to a multitude of nasty bacteria and they were wreaking havoc. In addition to the yeast infections, I was susceptible to every cold, flu, virus, and bug that was floating around. I was often sick and lethargic, dealing with sinus congestion, ear aches, excess mucous and other less common illnesses such as chicken pox and the mumps.

What I could not have possibly known at the time, and what nobody else seemed to understand, was that *all* of my symptoms were linked to the food I was feeding my body. I know this is a tough concept for people to appreciate because it's not widely accepted in traditional western medicine. But, if you stop and think for a moment, food is one of the foremost stimuli that we are exposed to on a daily, weekly, monthly, and yearly basis. As such, it stands to reason that what we put in our mouths has a huge impact on our overall health and wellness. We are what we eat! The right kind of food has the power to build us up, nourish every cell in our body, and promote robust health. On the flip side, the wrong kind of food can, over time, damage our organs, promote inflammation, increase our toxic load, and deprive our body of life-sustaining nutrients which, in turn, results in less than optimal function and the absolute certainty of illness.

It might be helpful to explain my diet during my childhood years to help you understand how inflammation begins and that illness doesn't necessarily stem from a diet solely consisting of fast food and junk food— although I did eat my fair share of both. I was born in the 60s, before fast food restaurants became ubiquitous. My mother primarily cooked everything from scratch. The highly refined and processed 'food-like' product industry was just starting to become more popular, and, as we moved into the 70s, these products would become more common in my family's kitchen as well.

To start, I was a formula-fed baby, which put me at a disadvantage because it robbed me of all the immune-boosting, health-promoting nutrients of breast milk and left me vulnerable to illness. As a youth, much of my diet consisted of starchy carbohydrates – essentially a standard North American diet. Breakfast was generally a cereal and, while it may have been Rice Crispies or Corn Flakes instead of some rainbow colored, artificially flavored cereal, it was still full of simple sugars and generally topped with a good heaping of brown sugar. Lunch was usually a sandwich (more starchy/refined carbohydrates), and dinner would be meat and potatoes. I thought corn was a vegetable. I recall snacking on sliced bananas smothered in brown sugar and milk. Another common snack was a sandwich, made from white bread, smothered in margarine and filled with brown sugar. Brown sugar was popular in my household and a staple in my diet. My mother was also a baker, and I recall often coming home after school to the wonderful smell of freshly baked cookies, homemade doughnuts, cream puffs, and other yummy, sugary treats, which I devoured with gusto.

In my tween years, I have a recollection of being fascinated by the 'cheese–like' food that you would squeeze out of a package, through a star-shaped hole, onto crackers. I'm not sure what that cheese was made of, but it was advertised heavily on TV and I had to have it. I didn't even particularly like it, but I was intrigued by the packaging and the novelty of it so, I ate it. We also had something called Carnation Instant Breakfast. It was a flavored powder you mixed with milk, an early version of a protein powder, I suppose. The commercials for Carnation Instant Breakfast were enticing and I wanted it so bad. Like the squeezable cheese, it didn't taste great, but I drank it anyway.

I don't remember fresh fruits and vegetables comprising a large part of my diet. Even the Saskatoon berries that we used to pick at the lake, which I *loved*, were not eaten on their own. They were baked into a pie or we would smother them in cream and brown sugar. One of the regular 'salads' my mother used to make was made of peeled and sliced apples mixed in sweetened whipped cream. It was delicious and one of my favorites, but I'm not sure it would count as a serving of fruit. I always ate mandarin oranges at Christmas and I do remember eating lettuce or cucumbers mixed with sour cream, but, again, we rarely ate veggies or fruits on their own as a regular part of our diet.

My food memories as I was growing up are mainly of dairy, lots of starchy simple carbohydrates, and *tons* of sugar. I drank pop (or as my American friends know it, soda), ate chocolate bars and other types of candy, and guzzled milk like it was water. Not unlike how many people eat today. Ann Wigmore said, "The food you eat can be either the safest and most powerful form of medicine or the slowest form of poison." My diet of wheat, sugar, and dairy was definitely the worst form of poison although it would take some time for me to figure this out.

Despite all of my health issues, my body was performing amazingly well. I had youth on my side! I was an avid figure skater, often skating five and six days a week all through the winter. In the summer, I was a competitive swimmer. I would train morning and night during the week and spend the weekends competing in meets around the province. I enjoyed both sports and managed to do well in school.

In Grade 12, I developed mononucleosis — this is caused by the Epstein Barr virus. This was a blow. It knocked me out for weeks. I was exhausted, lethargic, unable to walk from the family room to the kitchen without feeling wiped out. I missed several of my Grade 12 finals and my mom had to arrange for me to write these on alternate dates. I also had to pull out of the competitive swimming season because I just didn't have the energy or stamina to keep up with training. At the time, I had no idea that the mononucleosis was just another sign/symptom, in my long history of signs and symptoms, that my body was extremely unhappy. Mono was an obvious next step in the escalating signals my body was desperately trying to send me. But, again, nobody was listening.

Following graduation from high school, I got a job so I could start saving money. My goal was to backpack around the world. There was so much to see and do and I was determined to experience as much as I could. While I was certainly functional, I wasn't especially healthy. I was always fatigued, always struggling with gastrointestinal (GI) issues, and I was still getting tonsillitis. However, I persevered and continued to move forward towards my goal.

Finally, two years after graduation, when I was 19, the doctors said they needed to remove my tonsils. I was told they were so enlarged, inflamed, and nasty that they needed to come out. I was thrilled! Unfortunately, I had no idea that my tonsils were actually the sentinels of my immune system and I desperately needed to keep them. And, again, I had no idea that my repeated tonsillitis was my body telling me my immune system was malfunctioning and that I was actually severely inflamed. It was 1984, and I was just *so* happy to be getting rid of the offending organs that had plagued me mercilessly for the last 8 years. Good riddance was my sentiment!

Little did I know; my body was not done sending me signals about being unhappy just because I had my tonsils removed. The body is ingenious and persistent. It will find ways to express its unhappiness no matter what you do to ignore it.

● ● ●

CHAPTER 2
Ravaged

When diet is wrong medicine is of no use,
when diet is correct medicine is of no need
— AYURVEDIC PROVERB

When I was 20, I set off on my travels. I bought an open-ended ticket that would take me from Canada (Edmonton, Alberta, to be exact) to Fiji, Australia, New Zealand, the Cook Islands, and then back to Canada. I planned to be gone for one year. This was before the internet, so my only way to communicate with my family back home was through hand-written letters and payphones when I could find them. The trip was amazing. It was an education I could not have obtained anywhere else. I met so many different people and I experienced so many unique things. It truly was the trip of a lifetime. The only downside to the trip was that I struggled with some gastrointestinal symptoms on and off for the entire time I was away. I had lots of gas, bloating, and frequent bouts of diarrhea. I chalked this up to the food, the constant challenge of travel, and the different water. On the road, my lunch might be a Snickers bar. I often ate fast food. On occasion, when I would settle in somewhere for a few weeks, I would buy some groceries and cook for myself… but I wouldn't say I was eating full, home-cooked meals. Hostels and backpacking establishments are not equipped for gourmet cooking, so while I might scramble up some eggs with toast, toss a few salads, and perhaps throw some shrimps on the 'Barbie' with a few token vegetables, I was not consistently eating a regular whole foods diet.

I celebrated my 21st birthday in the Cook Islands and I returned home in the fall of my 21st year. It was September 1986. Upon returning home, my health seemed to stabilize as I found a job and got settled. I had spent a lot of money on my trip and needed to work two jobs in order to make up for lost income. I was busy working and trying to re-establish my social life. When people get busy, one of the first things that suffers is diet. I was no exception, eating on the run and grabbing food that is quick and easy means eating processed and refined food. My part-time evening job was as a server in a restaurant, so I was often eating restaurant food; things like potato skins, nachos, French fries, burgers, deep fried mozza sticks, French onion soup loaded with melted cheese, and the like.

Looking back, it's not a surprise that my health started to deteriorate again; the same symptoms I had when I was travel-ing resurfaced: gas, bloating, cramps, diarrhea. I went to see the doctor and was told I was simply burning the candle at both ends, I was too busy and stressed out, I needed to get more sleep; things would be fine. Back then, I trusted doctors. I thought they knew everything, I assumed they knew what was going on in my body. I had complete and total trust in what I was told.

I carried on and, sure enough, the symptoms subsided. Until they flared up again, that is. This became a consistent pattern for me over the next three years. The abdominal pain was, at times, excruciating. There were times I was afraid to leave the house in case I needed a bathroom. I often felt weak and dehydrated because I would be going to the bathroom 12-15 times a day, but every time I would go to the doctor the symptoms would be dismissed as a flu bug, too much fiber, not enough sleep, stress, anxiety, or a variety of other things.

The symptoms would come and go and, because the doctors didn't seem too concerned, I just started to think this was my 'normal'. I remember talking to my sister and explaining the pain I often experienced. I told her it felt like someone was twisting my intestine, like when you make a balloon animal. It felt like they were twisting and twisting and twisting until it felt like I was going to pass out from the pain and then it would be released and my gut would relax back in to its normal state. She looked at me, somewhat flabbergasted, and I recall her clearly saying, "that's not normal". I was a little surprised at this and thought to myself it "was" my normal.

During this time, I returned to school to get a diploma in Rehabilitation Studies. I planned to work with people who had developmental disabilities. I felt called to work in some kind of helping profession and the idea of helping people who were marginalized and disenfranchised resonated deeply for me. I wanted to advocate on their behalf and help them live full lives.

My schoolwork was intense. I found myself busy working a part-time job to help cover my expenses and managing a full class load at school. Once again, my gastrointestinal symptoms flared up but they didn't abate this time. I had constant abdominal pain and cramping, I was going to the bathroom upwards of 16 times per day, I was significantly dehydrated, I was burping like a truck driver, and I was exhausted from working and going to school.

As time went on, I knew instinctively that this was not stress, too much fiber, or not enough sleep. I *knew*, in fact I had known for a long time, that there was something seriously wrong. Given my challenges with getting the doctors to believe there was something wrong, I thought I needed to do some research and arm myself with information for when I did see the doctor. Once again, this was before the age of the internet, so, for my research,

I went to the library and started looking through medical books. I finally found a condition that seemed to fit my symptoms. It was Colitis. Armed with this information, I went to see the doctor and told him that I was positive I had Colitis and I was desperate for help. This time, the doctor agreed there was something amiss and I was referred to a gastroenterologist, a doctor who specializes in intestinal and digestive diseases.

There are often wait times to see specialists these days, but back in the 80s I was able to see him fairly quickly. My first visit with him was in the emergency room of the hospital where he was doing rounds. His name was Dr. Mario Milan. I clearly recall everything about that visit including what I was wearing. I explained my symptoms and he did an examination, I remember him asking me if I was always this pale. I didn't know it, but, at that point, I was highly anemic given the amount of blood I was losing in my stool. I am 5'8" and I weighed around 112lbs. I was not absorbing any nutrients from my food, everything was just passing right through me. The specialist wanted to do a barium enema to confirm his diagnosis. Following this unpleasant procedure, I saw him in his office and he told me I had Crohn's Disease. I was 24.

I have to say I was so happy to have a diagnosis for what I was experiencing. When you look relatively normal, people expect you to behave in a certain way, so it was such a relief to have a diagnosis that let people know I *was* sick; I wasn't faking it, I genuinely did not feel well. I was immediately started on heavy doses of corticosteroids which seemed to help minimize my GI symptoms. Unfortunately, every time I tried to start weaning down on the steroids, the disease would flare up again. I was still going to school full-time and working part–time; and I was still exhausted, anemic, and weak despite the pharmaceutical regime.

I was seeing Dr. Milan about once every two weeks. He was middle-aged, he wore glasses, and he was somewhat soft around the edges but I still developed a major crush on him. He definitely wasn't my type, so I'm not sure what triggered the crush. But, in hindsight, I think it had to do with the fact that he understood my symptoms. He believed me when I told him I had tremendous pain. He understood the intensity and urgency of my symptoms. And, he was able to make me feel better even if it was only temporary. I used to look forward to my visits with him, although I wasn't happy being on so many drugs. Each drug had a side effect and I didn't like this, so I would always try and negotiate with him. He would suggest I wean down on the steroids from 45mg/day to 40mg, and I would try and negotiate for 35mg. I have no doubt I pushed his patience to the max.

I think the worst side effects were from the steroids. Corticosteroids are nasty. While they may provide some immediate relief, their long-term use results in some very unpleasant side effects. They redistribute your body fat; they strip fat off your limbs and redeposit it on your trunk, often causing a swollen belly and something called a "buffalo hump" which is exactly what it sounds like, a big hump of tissue on your upper back. They also cause the face to swell up resulting in something called "moon face", it's either a result of more fat being distributed around the face or fluid retention, another unwanted side effect. Steroids can also cause excess body hair to grow in all the areas you don't want excess body hair. Mood swings, insomnia, jitters, weight gain, suppressed immune function, bone thinning, and acne are also typical side effects and all things I experienced while taking steroids. I look back and wonder at the logic that suggests you take a horrible drug that might manage one or two symptoms, but promotes and encourages a host of others that are equally damaging to the body. Unfortunately, this seems to be the basis for traditional western medicine. But, at that point in time, I was still at a stage in my life where I believed the doctor knew what was best for me and my health.

Ultimately, my symptoms were not responding to the steroids. Every time I started to wean off them, my symptoms would flare up, so Dr. Milan decided to hospitalize me so I could be fed intravenously and give my digestive tract a break from food. As with the diagnosis, I felt tremendous relief to be hospitalized. This allowed me an opportunity to just be sick. I could finally just rest. I didn't have to maintain a full caseload at school while working part-time. But, being in hospital is no fun. I was hooked up to a main line that fed me my nutrients. I was not allowed anything by mouth, and that was agonizing! Every commercial on TV is about food, and my mouth would water watching all those ads for pizza, burgers, deep-fried chicken and candy. I remember sneaking into the kitchen on my unit one day, scavenging for food. I found a bag of bread in the fridge and I stole a crust to eat. It tasted heavenly and luckily, it did not cause any gastrointestinal upset.

I was also being pumped full of drugs that had unpleasant side effects. I would often feel nauseous, or have a tinny taste in my mouth, or numbness in my hands and feet. I was miserable, but my symptoms were slowly becoming more manageable. I wasn't running to the bathroom 15 times a day and the pain in my gut was lessening.

After I was released from the hospital, I went home and tried to live my life. Around this time, my sister found a book called *"Food and the Gut Reaction"* by Elaine Gottschall. My sister had heard Elaine on a talk show and was impressed; she bought the book in the hopes it might help me. Gottschall was ahead of her time, and I wish I would have recognized the lifeline that her book provided me but, at the time, I was not ready to hear what she was suggesting.

The hallmark piece of *"Food and the Gut Reaction"* is the Specific Carbohydrate Diet — a diet based on the belief that certain foods impair gut function and leave it vulnerable to disease. She noted that poor diet repeatedly stresses the intestinal tract, resulting in progressive inflammation, malabsorption, nutritional

14

deficiencies, and the fast track to diseases such as Crohn's, colitis, IBS and diverticulitis. Her theory was that you could heal your digestive tract by following the Specific Carbohydrate Diet, which was essentially no grains, no added sugars, no milk (plain yogurt and aged cheeses were allowed), and no processed or refined foods.

When my sister presented this to me, I remember thinking "are you kidding me?". If I eliminated wheat, sugar, and dairy what was I going to eat? My sister made me soups, homemade yogurt, and a variety of other foods that were allowed on the Specific Carbohydrate Diet but I was 24 and not ready to make these changes. I was still clueless about how diet impacted the body and the doctors didn't seem to think my diet had a single thing to do with my illness, so why would I believe some crazy lady who wrote a book? If it was that easy to heal your digestive tract, then why wasn't everyone doing it and why weren't the doctors recommending it? If I had been more open and receptive, and if I had followed Ms. Gottschall's advice, I would have avoided a world of pain and hurt. But, at the time, I was not ready for this ground-breaking information. I was still going down the road recommended by my gastroenterologist: pharmaceuticals, pharmaceuticals, and more pharmaceuticals. And when that didn't work — surgery.

After my first hospitalization, I was feeling pretty good. I went back to school, returned to my job, and tried to get back into a routine. I was still taking medication, up to 32 pills per day, but my symptoms seemed to be well-managed. However, without any real change to the diet I was feeding my body, it was only a matter of time before my symptoms would flare up again. Every time my symptoms flared up I would go back on steroids. And when I would try to wean off the steroidal drugs, my symptoms would re-emerge. I would need to increase the dosage again or be hospitalized until things stabilized.

This was very trying on me and my family. I recall my dad sitting by my hospital bed one day telling me that he would give the world to trade places with me. I remember my sister spending the night at the hospital, sitting by me with her head resting on the edge of my bed. My brother was doing a residency in the same hospital where I was being admitted, and I have memories of him stopping by after rounds to review my chart and visit with me. My mom would spend most of her days at the hospital keeping me company, loving me and supporting me. It was a challenging time for my entire family, but it was reassuring to be surrounded by people who loved and cared for me.

About 18 months after my initial diagnosis, I started experiencing bowel obstructions. This happens due to a buildup of scar tissue in the intestines following repeated flare-ups. The tissue thickens up to the point that the bowel becomes obstructed. Due to the ongoing obstructions, I had a colonoscopy to see what was going on. I remember Dr. Milan telling me that there was a place in my small intestine, where it connects to the large intestine, and the opening was as big as the inside refill of a Bic pen. Typically, the digestive tract is about 1" in diameter. Mine was so scarred that the opening around the ileocecal valve (the joining of the small intestine to the large intestine) was no bigger than a pen refill. It was only a matter of time before surgical intervention was likely needed.

A few months after the colonoscopy, I had a fairly serious obstruction. I had been at my parent's cabin at the lake (Alberta Beach, AB) all day. We had a garage sale that day. The weather was gorgeous and it was warm and sunny. Around noon, I started experiencing intermittent pain in my gut. Every few hours, I would have about 30-40 minutes of intense pain. My sister said it reminded her of being in labor, but I was not pregnant. The pain would eventually subside, and I would go about my business for another few hours until the pain struck again. Near the end of the day, the time between the episodes of pain became shorter and shorter. The pain was exhausting, and we had all had a busy day hosting the garage sale.

I think we were all in bed by about 9:00pm, but the ongoing pain kept me awake. By this time, it was pretty much constant. I recall that around midnight my sister came to check on me, and when she saw the pain had not gone away she said I needed to get to the hospital. My dad drove me, I still remember he sped all the way and he went through multiple red lights. Luckily, we made it to the hospital in one piece. I was admitted and, because of the risk associated with bowel obstructions, I was referred to a surgeon. After some consultations, the decision was made to operate. Dr. Adams, my surgeon, talked to me about the risks, but, once again, I was so desperate to resolve my symptoms that I would have done anything.

Prepping for bowel surgery is *not* fun. You have to drink a significant amount of a foul-tasting liquid, in a short period of time, to clear out the bowel and ensure it is squeaky clean for surgery. Unfortunately, I was unable to gag down the liquid in a reasonable amount of time, so they had to stick a tube down my throat and pour the liquid into my stomach. Believe it or not, I was thrilled to have that tube down my throat because that meant I didn't have to taste that terrible bowel cleaning concoction.

I was still pretty young at this time and I had been living with debilitating symptoms, so I don't think I fully appreciated the gravity of having bowel surgery. I was just happy that something was going to happen to improve my health. My biggest concern was the massive scar I was going to have across my abdomen. The last thing I said to Dr. Adams before being put to sleep was "please leave my belly button intact — don't cut through my belly button". He said he would do his best and, sure enough, he made the incision below my belly button and left it intact. I was grateful for this.

Dr. Adams' resident, Dr. Daudi and my gastroenterologist, Dr. Milan, came to see me following the surgery and confirmed they had cut out two portions of my intestine as the disease had literally destroyed the tissue. They said they took out about 16 inches of my terminal ileum, including the ileocecal valve, which was severely scarred. The terminal ileum is the last piece of the small intestine and it plays a role in digestion and absorption of nutrients. It is also the only place in the body where vitamin B12 is absorbed, so I was told I would need B12 injections the rest of my life. The ileocecal valve is what separates the small intestine from the large; it releases digested food from the small intestine in to the large. The ileocecal valve also blocks these waste materials from backing up into the small intestine. It is intended to be a one-way valve, only opening up to allow processed foods to pass through. A fairly important gatekeeping job. Without an ileocecal valve, the toxic waste in my large intestine could back up into my small intestine and wreak havoc with my body. I didn't fully appreciate what that would mean for me later in life and how my intestinal health would suffer, significantly, as a consequence.

They also said they removed about 4 to 6 inches of my transverse colon due to significant scarring. The transverse colon is the longest region of the large intestine and is located between the ascending and descending colon. Most of the absorption and feces formation takes place in the transverse colon, making it a very important region of the digestive system. Once again, this was a vital piece of anatomy, critical to optimal digestive health, and it was gone from my body. To this day, I still experience fluctuations in my bowel function due to these missing body parts and I have to work diligently, on a daily basis, to maintain balance.

Following the surgery (my surgical report is included in the appendix at the end of the book), I was also told that the disease was quite severe and my entire digestive tract appeared to have lesions, so I would be sick the remainder of my life. This was not what a 25-year-old woman wanted to hear, but I was grateful that the sickest parts of my gut were gone and that perhaps I had a chance for reasonable health for a few years.

After I was discharged, I went to parents' house to recover. I was only going to take a few weeks off and then return to work because I didn't have disability insurance. But, my body had another plan in mind. I hadn't been at my parents' house too long, a few days at most, when I woke up one morning with a burning sensation in my abdomen. I had no idea what this was so I rolled over, took a painkiller, and tried to go back to sleep. I laid there for about an hour, but the pain just seemed to get worse. Not only did the pain get worse, but, when I tried to sit up and take another painkiller, I realized I was literally paralyzed. The pain was so intense I could not sit up. I could move my arms and legs, but other than that I was incapacitated.

I called for my mom and asked her to call my gastroenterologist for advice. Before she called him, she called my dad and, apparently, he said "Call the ambulance!". So, she called the ambulance first and then my gastroenterologist. The EMTs arrived almost immediately and loaded me onto a stretcher. The paramedic was able to speak to my gastroenterologist on the phone as they were wheeling me out; apparently, my GI said they shouldn't give me any painkillers as he didn't want to mask what was going on. My opinion was that I would have loved to mask what was going on but, unfortunately, I was overruled.

Back to the hospital I went; no speeding and no running red lights this time, though. They didn't even turn on the sirens. They told me my condition wasn't life–threatening, so they were going to go a nice, steady pace. When I arrived to the hospital, I spent most of the day in the ER. The ER doctors wanted to do a pelvic exam to try and figure out why I was having pain. They suggested that perhaps I had a ruptured ovarian cyst. I wanted to scream at them that the reason I had pain was because I had surgery 10 days before and something had gone seriously wrong. I knew this was no ruptured cyst, but I was weak and vulnerable and not in a position to advocate for myself. My sister, who was not at the hospital, was frantic. She was at home with her kids and calling the ER every few hours demanding to know if I had been seen by the surgeon who had done the surgery. Later on, my sister told me that the ER nurses were not pleased with her persistent follow-up. In fact, one of the nurses finally told her that she wasn't doing me any favors by bothering them and that they would not want to tend to me if she was going to continue being a thorn in their sides. My mother was with me, but she was from a generation that never questioned authority and she was certainly not going to question what was being done by the medical professionals. So, I continued to lay in ER while residents and nurses poked and prodded me and took my vital signs trying to figure out the cause of my pain.

Thank goodness, my sister wasn't willing to let a few harsh words from the ER nurse turn her off. She changed tack and called Dr. Adams' office directly. She was assertive enough that she ended up being transferred to my surgeon. When she finally got a hold of him, she said, "Do you know that one of your patients, whom you just operated on a few days ago, is in your ER?". He responded by saying he had just been told about it. My sister suggested he get down to see me asap and he said he was on his way. I was so relieved to see him. He immediately took charge and finally ordered something to kill the pain. After examining me, he surmised that one of the anastomoses (the place where he would have sewn the bowel together) had leaked and I had toxic bowel contents oozing into my abdomen. He told me they may have to do emergency surgery to remedy the situation and, if that was the case, I would need to wear a colostomy bag for a period of time following surgery. He said they would give me some anti-biotics and other medications and monitor the situation for a few hours before making that decision.

I was relieved that, within a few more hours, the pain started to subside and it appeared my body, with the help of the drugs he recommended, had been able to contain the leak and repair itself. Whew! I was so relieved I didn't need another surgery and that I wasn't going to have a colostomy. I spent another five days in the hospital recovering, and then went home to recuperate some more. It was at that point that I decided I would take the rest of the summer off work (about another twelve weeks) to give my body time to rest and repair. Although I didn't have private disability benefits, I was able to apply for sick benefits through the federal government. Given the status of my health, I was approved quickly after submitting the necessary paperwork and the supplemental income allowed me to take the necessary time to focus on my recovery.

I spent the next 3 months trying to reclaim some of my former function. I rested, read books, went for walks, and generally tried to rebuild my health. I also started to wean off the heavy duty drugs I had been taking for the last several years. I was able to get down to one maintenance drug that was supposed to minimize the risk of future flare ups. Over time, I was able to gain some strength and start to feel human again. But, my health issues were far from over.

● ● ●

CHAPTER 3

A Shift in Thinking

Natural forces within us are the true healers of disease
— HIPPOCRATES

During the next few years, I felt relatively good compared to what I had been dealing with prior to my surgery. While my gastrointestinal issues were greatly improved and I had stopped taking pharmaceuticals for the Crohn's disease, my general health was dismal. I struggled regularly with debilitating fatigue, swollen glands in my throat, sinus infections, and ear infections. My health still seemed to dictate what I could and couldn't do. I never felt energized; I never felt vibrant or robust. I always felt sickly. I thought that was my normal. I thought this was the way life would be for me. I always marveled at how other people seemed to be healthy and living their lives to the fullest. I wondered why everyone else was doing so well and I was struggling just to function on a daily basis.

Being sick can be socially isolating. You don't have energy to go out with friends or meet new people. And dating with an inflammatory bowel disease can be challenging. There is always the fear that you will have some kind of bowel spasm when you are out in public somewhere and you will need a bathroom immediately. Or, even worse, you might have an accident. This is not first date material and it can be uncomfortable trying to explain your needs to a potential suitor. It was during this difficult time that I met a man named Ric. We were set up by a friend and met on a blind date. I didn't know it on our first date, but I would later marry this man. Our first date was October 28, 1996; I was 31. As we started dating, I was up front about my health problems. He was very supportive and understanding. There were often times I could not do things because of my poor health and he always seemed to take this in stride. When we met, he had custody of his three daughters, so when we married on May 12, 1999, in Cancun, Mexico, I also became a stepmother to three wonderful girls.

In the early years of marriage, I struggled on and off with my symptoms; things would flare-up on occasion, but the flare-up would generally resolve fairly quickly without the use of hard core pharmaceuticals. However, we often missed events or social gatherings because I wasn't feeling well or didn't have the energy to go out. I was still getting ear infections and sinus infections and struggling with excess mucous and phlegm in the back of my throat. I would go to the doctor with my painful ears, and he would invariably diagnose an ear infection and prescribe antibiotics. I would always ask the doctor how he knew it wasn't viral and he would respond by saying he could just tell. He would say my ears were so red and inflamed that he recognized it as a bacterial infection needing medication. I was back to taking antibiotics 5-6 times per year for these supposed ear infections and I was still relying on the doctor to tell me what was best for my health and well-being.

I was also struggling on-and-off with bowel obstructions and ended up in the hospital a few times. These obstructions would eventually clear on their own without the use of drugs. The surgery had created more scar tissue, known as adhesions, on top of what was already there from repeated flare ups. So, my gut was struggling to function optimally and there was even the suggestion

I may require another surgery to cut through the adhesions as that may help manage the obstructions. Overall, I would have said I was healthy; but, in reality, I was still pretty sickly.

About a year before I got married, I decided to return to school so I could earn a degree. I went to the University of Calgary and graduated, with honors, with a Bachelor's Degree in Community Rehabilitation and Disability Studies. Despite my ongoing health problems, once I graduated, I found a job and started working full-time. I must admit, I always found it draining to work full-time and also deal with the myriad of health problems that continued to plague me, but I did my best not to miss work and to be a productive team member.

Every morning when my alarm went off, I would drag myself out of bed and get to work. Even though I always felt lousy, I never gave less than 110%. One of the things my parents had instilled in me was that you do what you have to do, it didn't really matter whether you wanted to or not, you just did it. I later learned that this was a limiting belief and that it doesn't necessarily serve your greater good to work yourself to the point where you collapse, but, at the time, I was still of the mindset that you go to work no matter what the cost. So that's what I continued to do.

I clearly remember waking up one morning and feeling awful, my glands were swollen, it hurt to swallow, and my ears were throbbing. I just wanted to stay in bed. I lay there thinking to myself, "Is this my life? Is this how I am going to live until I die?". I remember thinking I have done everything the doctors asked me to do, and I am still completely debilitated. I had to face the fact that I was always sick and tired and that if the disease didn't kill me, the treatment likely would. I knew I could *not* return to the doctor for another course of antibiotics *again*. I recalled an expression I had heard earlier. Something about the definition of insanity was doing the same thing over and over and expecting a different outcome. Well, I was done with insanity. I knew I had to try something different if I wanted to feel better.

That morning was a turning point for me. As I lay there wondering about the state of my health, I had a clear thought that there *had* to be another option. Intuitively, I realized I did not have to be sick and tired all the time. That morning, I decided I was going to take charge of my health and I was going to do something proactive to address my symptoms. I had reached my rock bottom. I was sick and tired of being sick and tired, and I was ready to do something about it!

When I arrived at work that morning, I pulled out the yellow pages (this was still in the days before the internet was readily available) and started looking up Naturopathic Doctors (ND). I had three criteria for finding a naturopath: 1) The office had to be in my quadrant of the city; 2) The person answering the phone had to be nice to me; and 3) The naturopath had to be able to see me that day. I think I found four or five ND's in the right part of the city, and I started calling them. I struck gold when I contacted Integrative Health and was able to schedule an appointment with Dr. Jeoff Drobot later that day.

I could not have known at the time but, Dr. Drobot was about to change my life. Dr. Drobot came from a family who believed whole heartedly in alternative, holistic health; his father was a naturopath, one of his sisters was a naturopath, and his other sister was a chiropractor. It was Dr. Drobot's first year in practice and that was probably the best thing that could have happened to me. He was fresh out of school and full of knowledge, he had lots of time to devote to his patients, and he was new enough to still be an idealist.

That first appointment lasted an hour and it was the most informative and enlightening medical appointment I had had to date. Dr. Drobot was able to connect all the dots for me; he was able to make sense of my history in a way no other doctor had been able to do. He explained that my body had been showing signs of inflammation from the time I was a little girl. The fact I had not been breast fed likely compromised my gastrointestinal health and left my gut vulnerable to threats. This, coupled with a pitiful diet made up primarily of wheat, sugar, and dairy, had been stressing my body for years. The years of canker sores, tonsillitis, ear infections, sinus infections, excess mucous, Crohn's disease; all signs of inflammation! My body had been communicating and sending me signals for years but, I did not understand the language.

By the time I saw Dr. Drobot, I was so desperate to get better that I would have done anything he suggested. I just wanted to reclaim some level of health and I had finally found someone who was making sense! He answered every question I had; he pieced together my entire history and he was able to logically explain what was going on in my body. No other doctor or specialist I had seen had been able to provide this level of insight. They all told me it was a 'mystery' why some people develop autoimmune conditions and others do not. Not one doctor *ever* looked back at my childhood problems and connected them to what I was experiencing as an adult. Not one doctor *ever* suggested that what I was eating could potentially be influencing my body. And not one doctor *ever* suggested I could do anything other than take drugs for my health. Finally, I was talking to someone who not only seemed to understand what was going on, but was also reassuring me that I could recover fully! My prayers were answered and I was committed to doing anything he recommended.

To my surprise, his recommendations were not outrageous and not difficult to achieve. Dr. Drobot asked me to cut out the three most common dietary allergens from my diet (wheat, sugar, and dairy) for three weeks. He said this would be enough time for my body to start regenerating. In my head, I questioned the simplicity of his advice. His advice was very similar to the suggestions from author Elaine Gotschall but, this time I was ready to make the change. The recommendations were totally achievable and I wondered how something so basic could actually make a difference but, I was willing to try. He also recommended some key supplements to rebuild my digestive tract and my immune system, both of which were decimated at this point in time. Driving home, I felt unbelievably optimistic. I was *full* of relief! Dr. Drobot had given me back my power. This information was an epiphany. Things that had been mysterious were all of a sudden clear. Questions that I had were now answered. Where there had been doubt, there now was clarity. That visit was a defining moment; it was an opportunity to start my life over.

● ● ●

CHAPTER 4

A New Beginning

Health is not simply the absence of sickness
— *HANNAH GREEN*

I was very excited to embark on my new dietary regime. There were definitely going to be challenges; back then, eating gluten free had not yet become fashionable and alternative milk options were limited. But, for the most part, I still had a lot of choice and I could almost eat anything and everything; this was going to be more about a lifestyle adjustment than restricting my food intake. And I obviously had to learn how to look at eating in an entirely new light. However, that wasn't very hard, given how quickly I started feeling better. It was fascinating to me that within the first three or four days of eliminating wheat, sugar, and dairy, I started to experience improvements. I didn't feel so crappy, I had fewer headaches, my throat wasn't sore, my glands didn't feel so swollen, my ears didn't hurt as much, and my gastrointestinal symptoms were improving. All this after only a few days.

Needless to say, at the end of three weeks, I was so blown away by what was happening in my body that I was more than willing to continue. With Dr. Drobot guiding me, I continued learning to eat real, whole foods versus processed and refined food. Every day was a new experience; I was shopping differently, I was scouring recipe books for inspiration, I was buying and cooking with foods I had not previously eaten, and I was revamping recipes that I had used in the past so they conformed to my new way of eating. My husband was somewhat skeptical and a little resistant, as might be expected. But, for the most part, he was a willing participant and when he started to see the positive results, he jumped on board completely.

The first year was a bit of a rollercoaster. I would feel great, and then I would allow wheat, dairy or sugar to creep back in and my symptoms would flare up again. It was a beautiful thing: my body would provide immediate feedback when I ate things that were not nourishing and nurturing. Having that instant response from my body was so helpful in keeping me on track; I was finally starting to get in touch with how I felt. I was learning to read the signs that my body was sending and understanding this form of communication.

As time went on, I started to get better at consistently eating wheat, sugar, and dairy free — something I was calling *clean eating*. I started to appreciate that once you eliminated these things, there was a whole world of choice available. As I became more consistent with my eating, my health continued to improve. After about two years of clean eating, I really started to experience a robust and vibrant level of health. I was not getting any colds or flus. My ear and sinus infections were gone. My throat was never sore. I had no more excess mucous or phlegm. I had increased energy. I was feeling better than I had felt in my entire life.

I had always loved traveling but, this can be difficult when you are dealing with a chronic illness. When I did travel I would usually come home sick and require one to two weeks of recovery to get back to normal. We had been married in May 1999, in Mexico, and one of the things we enjoyed doing was going back there for a week at an all-inclusive resort. With my newfound health, I was able to go to Mexico and indulge in an entire week of 'unclean' eating, with no detriments. Previously, if I had gone to Mexico for a week and indulged in wheat, sugar, dairy, and alcohol, I would have arrived home sick, congested, fatigued, and with an ear or sinus infection. Now I could go to Mexico (or anywhere else for that matter), enjoy myself, and not miss a beat when I arrived home. What progress!

In addition to my dietary changes, I started looking at some of my lifestyle choices and asking how I could do more to clean up my environment. I eliminated all chemical cleaners in the house, we installed a Reverse Osmosis machine in our kitchen so we could start drinking clean water, and whenever possible I opted for organic products. I started looking at my personal care routine as well and how I could reduce my exposure to all the chemicals that appeared to be ubiquitous in all personal care products. I was really starting to appreciate the value of clean living, not just clean eating.

●　●　●

CHAPTER 5

You Can't Please Everyone

A man too busy to take care of his health is like
a mechanic too busy to take care of his tools
— SPANISH PROVERB

Over time, I learned more and more. I read books and I also made it a point to follow certain holistic practitioners online like Food Matters, Dr. Mercola, and Josh Axe. Every day I was gaining more knowledge on how to support my health from the inside out.

My extended family had also started to make changes based on the new-found health I was experiencing. Family and friends were coming to me and asking advice about how to improve their health. My sister had struggled for years with a nail fungus. She had been to specialists who had offered a variety of pharmaceuticals which didn't help. She had tried rubbing garlic on her nails, massaging coconut oil or oil of oregano into her nails but nothing seemed to help. However, she noticed that the fungus would always clear up while she was on vacation in Mexico. She wasn't sure what it was about Mexico that was helping her nails. The humidity? Perhaps the sunshine? The salt water? When I started talking about the detrimental effects of consuming dairy, she finally made the connection that, while in Mexico, she wasn't drinking milk. When she arrived back to Canada, she experimented by eliminating cow dairy. The result? Perfectly clear nails. No more fungus.

Our middle daughter had a baby girl in 2008. Our new granddaughter struggled with skin issues and eczema from the day she was born. Our daughter tried a number of herbal and natural topical remedies and managed the skin issues quite well for a time. But, eventually, as our granddaughter got older and transitioned from formula to regular milk, the eczema exploded. It wasn't unusual to see this beautiful little girl's face covered in a nasty red rash.

Our daughter finally met with Dr. Drobot who suggested taking the toddler off wheat and dairy. The change was extraordinary. Within a few weeks, her skin had cleared up completely. All because of a change in diet. This was one of the most obvious examples of the old adage "we are what we eat." Not everyone was convinced though. Our daughter's in-laws were somewhat skeptical and believed that it was likely just coincidence that our granddaughter's skin cleared up so well after removing wheat and dairy from her diet. That year at Christmas, while the in-laws were babysitting, someone gave our granddaughter some Christmas baking. Apparently, she developed a rash around her mouth immediately, a clear indicator there was a definite connection between her diet and the skin issues. Needless to say, our daughter's in-laws are now on board and don't question the need for our granddaughter to avoid wheat.

My niece told me once that she had some skin issues. It wasn't anything major, but she said she noticed some dry, discolored, scaly skin around her armpits and on her lower abdomen. It wasn't overly concerning. What was interesting is that when she cut out wheat, sugar, and dairy, the skin totally cleared up. Years later, when she was pregnant with twins and her food cravings were leading her to eat more pizza, bread, and cheese, those same skin issues came back immediately. The human body is so amazing. It started communicating its unhappiness right away and my niece understood this language. She cleaned up her diet, and her skin cleared up immediately.

Our oldest daughter has always struggled with dairy; she experiences severe gastrointestinal upset when she consumes any type of dairy product. Based on her personal experience, she chose not to give her children dairy. I was in full support of this choice, but the public health nurse actually told her she was risking the development of her children by *not* giving them milk! This is so far from the truth, but it clearly illustrates that the misconceptions about the need for dairy are not restricted to the average person. Even our medical professionals are confused about certain foods and how what we eat can have a negative impact on our health.

While many of my family and friends were embracing the idea of clean eating, there were others who thought I was irrational. It was interesting to me how many people questioned what I was doing. People would actually debate with me about some of the choices I was making or advocating. What was even more interesting to me was that most of the people who would challenge me were sick. They were unhealthy and yet, wanted to argue the merits of the diet I was following. And there were also people who thought I had lost my mind. People who thought I was completely out of touch. People who just could not wrap their head around the concept that food could actually be medicine.

Even some of my lifestyles choices were being questioned. Early in 2010, there was a bad outbreak of H1N1 in the city where I lived. The provincial health care services branch of the government was advocating for a special flu shot to protect against this particular strain. I was not overly concerned and had no intention of getting a flu shot. No one in my immediate family was planning on getting a flu shot, either. However, the rest of the city was on high alert due to the fear campaign that was being waged by health care professionals threatening death and doom if you did *not* get vaccinated. People were swarming to the injection facilities and standing in line for hours so they could be 'protected.' I, on the other hand, was relying on my immune system to provide all the protection I needed.

At that time, we had a three-month-old granddaughter in our family. When some of our friends found out we had no intention of getting vaccinated, I was actually told I was putting my granddaughter's health at risk. A well-meaning friend told me that for my granddaughter's sake I should be vaccinated so I wouldn't infect her. I realized then how deeply some of our beliefs about health are ingrained. We have been brainwashed by the traditional allopathic medical model to believe that mainstream is the *only* way to go, and anything outside of this model is quackery. And, yet, this 'quackery' had saved my life and I believed wholeheartedly that I was on the right path and I would not be deterred by ignorance.

● ● ●

CHAPTER 6

Following my Passion

Our bodies are our gardens; our wills are our gardeners
— WILLIAM SHAKESPEARE

During the time I started my more holistic approach to health, I was working in the human service field providing support to people with developmental disabilities. As I mentioned earlier, I had gone back to university and earned a Bachelor's of Community Rehabilitation and Disability Studies, so I was now utilizing that degree by working as a manager for an organization that provided residential and vocational services to adults with developmental disabilities. I worked in an environment where I was exposed to sick people every day; we were providing support to 100s of adults whose health was compromised for a variety of reasons. Even though I was in management, I often spent time working directly with the individuals we served; I would assist them at meal times, I provided personal care, I cleaned up urine, feces and vomit, I performed transfers, or just offered comfort. Interestingly enough, as my immune system became stronger and stronger, I would never get sick. Waves of colds or flus would sweep through the building and I was immune! I never missed a day of work because I was never sick.

I eventually moved into a different role within the insurance industry, as a Rehabilitation Consultant. In this role, I worked with people who were on short-term or long-term disability and developed plans to help them return to work. My entire career was focused on helping people, but I dreamed of helping people as a Holistic Practitioner. Over the years, I checked online for various courses and programs that might allow me to work as an herbalist, an iridologist, an acupuncturist or something similar. But nothing really clicked until one day in 2013 when I was searching for something related to nutritionist, and I came across the Canadian School of Natural Nutrition (CSNN).

CSNN had been around for over 20 years at that time, but, for whatever reason, I had not discovered it in previous searches. Perhaps I had not been ready in previous searches, but, in 2013, I was clearly ready. I sent away for some of their literature and started reading about their 10 month Certified Holistic Nutritionist program. The more I read, the more I came to realize that this was exactly what I was supposed to be doing. This is what I had been looking for; this program felt like a great fit for me and would allow me to marry my passion for clean eating with an actual vocation that could earn me money! I attended an information session and registered immediately to start in the fall of 2014.

Before I even started school, I began dreaming of my own holistic nutrition consulting business. My husband and I would talk about it endlessly, discussing names, the types of services I would offer, ways to market my business and where I would work. This was an exciting time, it felt like I was about to embark on a new chapter in my life. One where I would be able to offer concrete help and support to people who were sick. I envisioned being able to offer my clients an alternative to the traditional; I dreamed of helping people reclaim their health and supporting them to live their life to the fullest. Given my personal experience, I felt strongly that this was my purpose in life.

I started school on August 25th, 2014. I remember being filled with anticipatory anxiety and excitement, and I was not disappointed! Every minute of every class was exactly what I had been looking for. I was learning new things every day and discovering new ways to support my health. Each day in school was exciting, exhilarating, and stimulating. Every day I would come home from class ready to change something in our routine; we were going to start taking a specific supplement, or we were going to start cooking with coconut oil instead of olive oil, or we were going to start chewing our food better, or we were going to start food combining, or we were going to start juicing... the list went on. The more I learned, the more changes we started to make. Lucky for me, my husband took all of these changes in stride and supported me every moment of every day and welcomed these changes with appreciation.

Early in October, I attended a workshop the school was offering on cooking with whole foods. It was an amazing day. I was with people who shared my enthusiasm for real food and nutrition. The instructors were speaking a language I understood. The other students weren't looking at me like I had two heads. I truly felt like I had found my home. When the day was over, I went to my car and cried tears of joy. I had finally found my people; a place where my views and ideas were not frowned upon, a place where the people around me shared my passions and beliefs. Nobody in that group was going to tell me I was risking the health of my granddaughter because I chose not to get a flu vaccination. I felt so empowered.

When I began school, I already felt like I had a basic understanding of diet and nutrition and how the body responds to food, but I could never have dreamed how much more information there was to learn. I was attending classes on pathology, anatomy, preventive nutrition, allergies, detoxification, cancer, eco-nutrition, pediatric nutrition, perspectives on aging, sports nutrition, alternative diets, pharmaceuticals, and symptomatology; we even attended a cadaver lab! I was stunned by what I was learning. The classes were really helping me understand some of the "whys" behind how the body responds to what we eat. I was hungry for this knowledge and I was soaking up every last detail with passion.

I eventually graduated, with honors, in September of 2015 and immediately started my own consulting practice. As I started to work with clients, I began to see firsthand that the majority of people are not thriving or living vibrant, robust healthy lives. I also started to meet clients who had Inflammatory Bowel Disease (Crohn's or Ulcerative Colitis) and they were struggling to manage their symptoms. I had several clients with inflammatory bowel disease tell me that the foods they had been told to eat were foods such as white bread, white rice, ice cream, puddings, and milkshakes. I was dumbfounded. I couldn't believe that the traditional allopathic medical model was still recommending the exact same foods they had recommended to me 25 years ago! The same foods that had essentially created the illness in my body! Despite all the progress that had been made in medicine over the years, it appeared that traditional medicine had still not learned anything about food and the impact it has on the body.

Shortly after I started working as a Holistic Nutrition Consultant, I had another turning point just like the one I had that morning about 20 years earlier when I woke up and knew that I was going to take charge of my health. This time, I woke up and realized that I needed to write a book. I wanted to share my journey with other people who were struggling with their health. I was meeting people who had the exact same condition as me, only they were sick and debilitated and I was living a vibrant, robust, and healthy life. I was hearing about people with inflammatory bowel disease who were dying and I knew this didn't have to happen. It had been 20 years since I had a sign or symptoms of Crohn's disease and I felt it was important to share what I knew in the hopes that it could help people reclaim their health.

As I started thinking about writing a book, I realized that there is a fabulous "Life After Crohn's" and that, in my opinion, total health and wellness essentially comes down to five basic steps. It is not rocket science. It is based on the premise that the body is an amazing machine and has an innate ability to perform efficiently, without illness, when you give it what it needs. My hope is for you to use the following pages as inspiration and motivation but, also as a guide or a template that will allow you to take back your own power and move forward on a journey towards vibrant health.

● ● ●

Part II – 5 Steps to Total Wellness

CHAPTER 7

Step I: Reduce Inflammation

*You can't afford to get sick and you can't depend
on the present health care system to keep you
well. It's up to you to protect and maintain your
body's innate capacity for health and healing
by making the right choice in how you live*
— ANDREW WEIL

Given that Crohn's disease is categorized as an inflammatory bowel disease, it stands to reason that the number one step to eradicating it starts with reducing inflammation. We have all heard the term inflammation, but what does it really mean? Inflammation is actually a normal and healthy response in the body. When you get an infection, inflammation is necessary to help protect and heal your body. During an inflammatory response, there are a series of biochemical reactions which mobilize white blood cells and other chemicals which are then dispatched to the injured area to fight off foreign invaders.

Think about an experience where you have cut yourself, picked up a sliver, or acquired some type of infection. The injured area typically becomes red, warm, swollen, and somewhat painful. This is a healthy and lifesaving response. Unfortunately, in today's world, we are seeing more and more *chronic* inflammation and this is not a normal or healthy process.

Chronic inflammation is a slow and insidious process whereby the body is undergoing countless assaults on a daily basis. It's not an infection, it's not a sliver, it's not a cut; it's a continuous onslaught of minor attacks or assaults day in, day out. These attacks build up over time and start to create an environment of inflammation (I'll explain more about what constitutes these attacks shortly). Slowly, this inflammation starts to work its way throughout the body until it ultimately becomes systemic, damaging various body systems. We now know that most chronic conditions are rooted in inflammation. My condition, Crohn's disease, is an inflammation of the digestive tract. Asthma is inflammation in the respiratory tract. Anklosing Spondylitis is inflammation in the spinal cord. Arthritis is inflammation of the joints. You get the picture. The bottom line is you cannot have "unwellness" in the body without systemic inflammation.

We all experience signs and symptoms of inflammation without understanding it. I have no doubt that every single person in North America has some level of inflammation in their body. It's shocking how many people assume their inflammatory symptoms are normal and just a part of life. In my case, I struggled for years with tonsillitis, canker sores, ear infections, sinus infections, mononucleosis, excess phlegm, and mucous. These are *all* signs of inflammation and if I had recognized this and taken steps to reduce the inflammation in my body, I likely could have avoided it from progressing to Crohn's disease.

What is causing this widespread inflammation? I believe chronic inflammation is the result of the daily assaults I mentioned earlier. You may be asking, "What constitutes an assault?". The answer is that our lifestyle is full of things that assault our bodies — smoking, environmental toxins, lack of sleep, stress, dehydration, a sedentary lifestyle, alcohol, and a poor diet, to name a few. For the purposes of this chapter, I am going to focus primarily on our dietary choices because I believe this is one of easiest and most important areas we can address to reduce chronic inflammation.

When I first went to the naturopath 20 years ago, he asked me to eliminate three things from my diet: wheat, sugar, and dairy. Why these particular foods? The answer is that they are likely the most common substances we ingest and the most inflammatory to the body.

Cow dairy is the number one allergen in the world! In North America, we have the highest incidence rate of osteoporosis despite the fact that we are also the biggest consumers of milk. This seems somewhat contradictory given we have been told repeatedly that we require milk for strong and healthy bones. Unfortunately, what we haven't been told is that once milk has been pasteurized it is essentially devoid of nutrients and what nutrients are left are not bioavailable to humans. It is important to note I am talking about pasteurized milk, *not* raw cow's milk. In fact, raw milk is actually very good for us. It contains all of its original fatty acids, vitamins, minerals, and phytonutrients, including phosphatase, an enzyme that aids and assists in the absorption of calcium in to your bones. Unfortunately, all of these health promoting nutrients are lost in the pasteurization process.

It's stunning to think that North Americans drink gallons of pasteurized milk but are not able to actually benefit from it. When I first started researching the dangers of cow dairy and discovered that we can't actually absorb the calcium in processed cow's milk, it was a revelation. Not only do we not absorb the calcium, we actually end up excreting more calcium when consuming cow dairy due to the high levels of phosphorus in the milk. In addition, cow's milk is virtually impossible for humans to digest; we do not produce the enzymes necessary to properly break down the protein in cow's milk. So, when the body is spending all its time trying to digest the constant 'assault' of cow dairy, it can't focus on other important jobs such as immune function, blood purification, or balancing of hormones to name a few.

I grew up guzzling milk from the carton. I *loved* my milk. I drank milk as a snack. I didn't think I could live without milk. But, when I found out it was causing inflammation in my body, that it was not providing any nutrition and my body was feeling much better without it, it was not a difficult choice to simply eliminate it. There are so many non-dairy alternatives available these days it's not a hardship. If you're worried about where you will get your calcium, a handful of almonds offers a better bio-available source of calcium than a cup of milk.

What about wheat and gluten? The multinational food manufacturers would have us believe that "whole wheat" is a healthy choice. The findings of the various research I have done is not in keeping with this information. In fact, what I have read indicates that the wheat today is so far removed from what we were eating in the 60s and 70s that our bodies don't even recognize it as food. Dr. David Perlmutter, author of Grain Brain, writes that while wheat is not genetically modified, it has been hybridized which means it's crossbred with other grains and species to produce a higher yield, *but* it also contains less nutrients and *more* carbohydrates. It's also important to remember the multinational corporations that dominate the agricultural food industry (from seed to shelf) are more interested in profit than in taste, selection, and nutrient density. It's called deliberate selection. The focus of conventional farming is yield (pounds per acre), size, resistance to disease, and heat tolerance. Nutrition, flavor, and health are not even a consideration in the business of wheat farming.

The most up to date literature tells us that the carbohydrates in modern wheat are so high that they raise blood sugar levels more than any other carbohydrate, including a candy bar! Gluten, a protein found in wheat, has been modified to a *super* gluten, double the gluten of its more natural cousin. Given this information, it's no wonder that celiac disease, a gluten allergy, has grown exponentially. But, I have come to learn that even if you don't have an actual gluten allergy, everyone is struggling with gluten sensitivities. There is even a substance in wheat called phytic acid which can bind minerals like calcium, zinc, iron, and magnesium in the body and prevent them from being absorbed. These are vital nutrients to our health and yet, if we are consuming excess wheat, we are not likely absorbing them.

There is also a whole school of research that outlines how gluten can actually damage the gut lining leading to a myriad of problems including, you guessed it, chronic inflammation. And an imbalance in our gut health is also linked to mental health disorders, migraines, joint pain, IBS, fatigue, skin-related issues, Candida, and brain fog. Along with dairy, wheat had been a staple in my diet! I loved bread, pasta, crackers, cookies, muffins, and bagels. But, every time I ate these things, I was essentially promoting inflammation. In hindsight, now that I understand the dangers of excess wheat consumption, it's no surprise my body developed Crohn's disease. But, even being wheat and gluten free doesn't mean I have to deprive myself. As with milk, there are numerous alternatives that taste good and won't compromise your gut health. I rarely eat refined grains but, when I am craving pasta I opt for a brown rice or kamut pasta. When I want a piece of toast I reach for spelt bread or a sprouted ancient grain bread. I even bake on occasion using buckwheat, spelt, coconut or almond flour. The choices are endless. It just requires a willingness to change.

That brings us to sugar. There is not one scrap of information anywhere that says sugar is healthy. Unless, of course, it's written by the sugar producers. Refined white sugar is what I consider an anti-nutrient, and is essentially toxic and highly inflammatory to the body. It has been stripped of all nutrients and it comes from sugar beets which are genetically modified. Did you know sugar stimulates the same neural pathways in the brain as cocaine, meaning it's addictive? Giving children cocaine on a daily basis sounds ludicrous, but all products geared towards children are laden with sugar. Most children, and most adults, are getting multiple 'hits' of this addictive substance every day.

Through a tremendous amount of reading, I have come to understand that sugar weakens the immune system, is highly acidic, and promotes inflammation. You might also be surprised to know that excess blood sugars get stored as adipose tissue around the waist (hello obesity) and it leads to a thinning of the bone because it strips calcium from the bones to help alkalize the blood when blood sugars are high, perhaps another factor in North America's high incidence of osteoporosis. Sugar also burdens the liver which can contribute to high cholesterol levels. Our society has demonized saturated fats for raising cholesterol, but I think fat may be the least of our worries. It's sugar that's killing us.

Another serious risk to our health is that sugar raises cortisol levels, creating a fight-or-flight response in the body which is linked to chronic and systemic inflammation. High cortisol also stresses the liver and pancreas and ultimately increases our cravings for sugar. The blood sugar rollercoaster most people experience on a daily basis results in things such as low energy, irritability, anxiety, negative moods, decreased focus, and concentration, along with a plethora of other symptoms. Sound familiar?

Sugar is known by about 60 different names. The food manu-facturers are trying to trick us into thinking there isn't any added sugar in their product by calling it by some other name. It's important to understand that things like malt, dextrose, dextran, carob syrup, lactose, maltose, and fructose are all other names for sugar. And artificial sweeteners, like aspartame and sucralose, are no better! Studies show that people who consume artificially sweetened drinks lose *less* weight than those who drink the same sugar sweetened version. How is this possible you ask? Artificial sweeteners change your gut bacteria and we know that diverse and healthy gut bacteria is critical to our overall health and well-ness, including maintaining our weight.

The average Canadian adult eats 26 teaspoons of sugar each day which equates to 104 grams (1 tsp = 4 grams). The World Health Organization recommends no more than 25g/day *total* for an adult. Which, in my opinion, is still much too high. A can of regular cola has 39 grams, 1 cup of regular almond milk (not the unsweetened) has 15 grams of sugar (over 3 tsp), and some granola bars have between 12 and 16 grams. We must eliminate refined sugar if we want to reduce inflammation in the body.

The good news is that eating 'sugar' free does not mean depriving yourself of sweet treats. There are so many other options available to us that provide some level of nutrition that we won't even miss the sugar. Options like dates, unpasteurized honey, blackstrap molasses, whole cane sugar, coconut palm sugar, and pure maple syrup are less inflammatory and much better choices for the body. I recently led a seven day sugar-free challenge on Facebook because I wanted to show people that clean eating does not mean you have to give up treats. Every day I posted yummy recipes that were sweetened with nothing more than bananas and dates. I received rave reviews, even from the hardcore doubters. It really is that easy. You just have to give it a chance and let your taste buds adjust to your new version of sweet.

Eliminating wheat, sugar, and dairy are three simple and very powerful steps that will deliver exponential benefits to the body. However, if you want to take things to the next level, let's talk about some other dietary changes that will go a long way towards further reducing inflammation in the body.

Healthy fats are unbelievably good for the body. Good fat helps stabilize blood sugar levels, it ensures we can absorb and utilize fat soluble vitamins such as, A, D, and E, it is very neuro-protective, and helps keep our brain functioning at optimal levels. Good fat helps manage appetite, decreases intense food cravings, and supports our immune system. We need good, healthy fats in our diet. What we don't need are trans fats and hydrogenated fats. Unfortunately, these 'bad' fats have become ubiquitous in processed and refined food today.

Trans and hydrogenated fats are actually damaging to our body and they are implicated in numerous serious health conditions. Trans and hydrogenated fats are free radicals (I'll talk more about free radicals in Chapter 10); they have been molecularly altered through the heating and refining process. Once ingested, they promote inflammation, they interfere with basic cell membrane function, they displace good fat, and generally wreak havoc anywhere and everywhere. This damage can pave the way for cancer, diabetes, neurological conditions (trans fats have an affinity for brain tissue), and cardiovascular dysfunction. Trans fats and hydrogenated oils are in the vast majority of processed foods, including crackers, chips, margarine, cake mixes and frostings, pancake and waffle mixes, non-dairy creamers, microwave popcorn, packaged cookies, blended creamy drinks, many packaged crackers, prepared puddings, and fried foods. It's quite the list, I know. If you want to reduce inflammation in the body, you want to avoid these nasty fats like the plague and focus more on healthy fats that come from avocados, nuts, seeds, organic butter, coconut oil, and organic meats and fish. Food additives are also highly inflammatory. When I talk about food additives, I am talking about the long list of unpronounceable ingredients on the side of every box, package, and container of manufactured food. Food additives are nothing more than chemicals that add to our overall toxic load and create inflammation in the body. Food dyes are a common additive found in cake mixes, relish, pickles, chewing gum, puddings, mac and cheese, jams and jellies, margarine and colored cereals and, are generally recognized as known carcinogens. If you are not familiar with carcinogens, they are defined as any substance or agent that can cause cancer. One of the most ubiquitous food dyes, Tartrazine (yellow #5), has been banned in several European countries due to its highly toxic effects on the body. Yet, in North America, it is still found in relish, mac and cheese, those little fish-shaped crackers, mustard, and even in some children's products such as colored fizzy bath tablets. BHA and BHT are other highly inflammatory chemicals that affect the nervous system and can cause behavioral issues in children. These are also banned in the UK, but are often found in cereals, instant potato flakes, frozen dinners, margarine, fruit drinks, lard, and baked goods in North America. Reading labels can actually save your life!

Another highly toxic, inflammation promoting and readily available additive is aspartame. Interestingly enough, more lawsuits have been launched against aspartame than any other artificial sweetener on the market. The recommended limit of aspartame is 7.9mg/day. A one-liter diet pop contains approximately 56mg of aspartame, that's more than seven times the recommended daily intake! And it's likely that some individuals are drinking more than 1 liter of pop per day. These toxins are being ingested by millions of people, in significant amounts, on a daily basis. The long-term cumulative effects of these compounds are staggering and, in my mind, partially to blame for the epidemic health crisis we are currently seeing nationwide. Reducing our exposure to these toxic food additives is critical. Start be reading every label and avoiding ingredients you can't pronounce. A better option would be to stop buying manufactured food and focus on eating a whole foods diet.

Identifying and eliminating food sensitivities is also critical to reducing inflammation. According to Dr. Mercola (mercola.com), food allergies are the fifth leading cause of chronic illness in the US — and their incidence is on the rise. When our body becomes sensitive to a particular food, it can cause a myriad of problems when we consume it. It is different from an actual allergy because, with an allergy, our body responds immediately with acute symptoms such as hives or anaphylaxis. With a food sensitivity, the response can take up to four days before we see a symptom. Food sensitivities wreak havoc in the body causing things like runny nose, migraines, excess mucous or phlegm, canker sores, cold sores, tonsillitis, sinus infections, ear infections, eczema and even bed wetting, which are all signs of inflammation in the body. Food sensitivity testing is becoming more and more widely available. If you have signs of inflammation in the body, even after you have eliminated the most common allergens, you may want to consider testing for food sensitivities so you can further support your health.

In my opinion, reducing inflammation in the body is the single most important step you can take towards improving your physical health. It has multiple benefits that will support *all* the systems of the body and allow you to start reclaiming some of what you have lost.

● ● ●

CHAPTER 8

Step II: Revise Your Diet

> *We can make a commitment to promote vegetables*
> *and fruits and whole grains on every part of every*
> *menu. We can emphasize quality over quantity.*
> *And we can help create a culture where our kids*
> *ask for healthy options instead of resisting them*
> — MICHELLE OBAMA

The quote by Ann Wigmore says it all: "The food you eat can be either the safest and most powerful form of medicine or the slowest form of poison". Truer words were never spoken. We are exposed to food multiple times per day, day after day, week after week, month after month, and year after year. It is an enormous component of our lives. As such, it is imperative that what we put in our mouths is nourishing and beneficial to the body. Each bite should be building us up. We must focus on a whole foods diet; that is, preparing your own food from ingredients that are as close to nature as possible. Think real food like fruits, vegetables, nuts, seeds, eggs, legumes, beans, whole grains, and organic meats, fish, and poultry.

For the majority of people, a whole foods diet really requires a shift in thinking from expediency to sustenance. Our society has really become dependent on manufactured food because of the convenience and ease that it offers. For breakfast, when everyone is rushing to get out the door on time, kids, and perhaps some adults, tend to scarf down a bowl of rainbow-colored cereal, a waffle out of a box, or a big, doughy bagel smothered in cream cheese. Lunch is often a sandwich, perhaps a pizza, or maybe a microwaveable low-fat option eaten while working at a desk. And supper is no different. Parents are getting home late from work, kids are hurrying off to dance class, soccer practice, or piano lessons, so the meal needs to be quick and easy. I think that's why families often choose to get their nourishment from a drive-through window or some fast and easy meal from a box. While this type of lifestyle may appear to be time saving, in the long run it will actually steal time from you. Being sick takes a tremendous amount of time and it robs you of your freedom. I spent countless days in hospital, I missed numerous events and activities because I was weak and tired, I lost income because I was too sick to work, and I missed half my life because I was too unwell to participate. In hindsight, I would have preferred to spend more time preparing nutrient-dense meals so that I could enjoy my life rather than spending it in a debilitated state.

It's imperative we start teaching our kids about nutrition and healthy eating when they are young. If I had understood the importance of a nutrient-dense diet and that what I put in my mouth is reflected in my overall health and wellness, I may have made different choices and perhaps avoided developing Crohn's disease. Unfortunately, it doesn't appear that kids are any more informed today about healthy eating than they were when I was growing up. In fact, it seems our kids today have become seriously disconnected from food. A recent survey I read out of Australia noted that one in five primary school children couldn't say where fresh food came from; one in four didn't know that butter comes from cow's milk; that apples and bananas are grown on trees; that potatoes are grown underground; or that tomatoes are grown on vines.

In my mind, this is a travesty. How are these children going to learn how to eat a nutrient-dense diet if they don't even know where their food comes from? It's critical to spend more time in the kitchen, with our kids, connecting them to food and teaching them about the importance of eating real food. If we don't take the time to do this now, there is no doubt that our children will struggle with health and potentially develop serious life-threatening medical conditions later in life. The other morning, I was in a hotel in St. George, Utah. There was a free breakfast included and while I can't usually find anything I want to eat in this type of environment I was passing through the dining room so I could get hot water for my tea. I walked by a table with a mother and her 3 sons. One of the boys had a plate full of donuts for breakfast and the other 2 boys each had a bowl of brightly colored O's drowning in milk. Perhaps this was not a typical breakfast for this family but it was discouraging for me to see it. There was a not a scrap of real food in sight and it is frightening to think that our children, who are still growing and developing, are not getting the nutrients they require to grow up strong and healthy.

In addition to eliminating the various foods mentioned in the previous chapter, I try to make sure my diet is organic as much as possible. I am often asked if there is really a difference between conventionally farmed food and organic. Let's consider the tomato as an example. 100 grams of today's fresh tomato compared to 100 grams of fresh tomato in 1963 contains:

- 30.7% less Vitamin A;
- 16.9% less Vitamin C;
- 61.5% less calcium;
- 11.1% less phosphorus;
- 9% less potassium;
- 8% less niacin; and
- 10% less iron.

This is a substantial loss in nutrients. But, it's not all about losses; in fact, there are two nutrients that have increased — the amount of fat in the tomatoes has increased by a whopping 65%, while sodium (the basis of common table salt) has increased by an astounding 200% (sourced from *The End of Food; How the Food Industry is Destroying our Food* by Pawlick, Thomas). The average conventionally farmed tomato is higher in fat and sodium, but lower in calcium, potassium, vitamin A, Vitamin C, iron, phosphorus, and niacin. Crazy, no?

You may wonder how on earth this can happen. It's called deliberate selection. Just like I talked about with the hybridization of wheat, the multinational corporations that dominate the agricultural food industry (from seed to shelf) are more interested in profit than they are in taste, selection, and nutrient density. The focus of conventional farming is yield (pounds per acre), size, resistance to disease, heat tolerance, uniformity of shape, and uniformity of ripening. The top two characteristics that most consumers are looking for, flavor and nutritional content, are not even a consideration.

Aside from the superior nutritional content of organic produce, we should also consider the toxic load of the many herbicides and insecticides that are used in conventional farming. Many herbicides and pesticides are known carcinogens, inflammatory to the body, and they are also endocrine disrupters, meaning they mess with our hormones. Our bodies would do so much better if they were not being continually exposed to these toxic chemicals.

In some instances, organic fruits and vegetables can cost more than their conventionally farmed counterparts. So, in the interest of economics, download the Dirty Dozen/Clean Fifteen app from The Environmental Working Group. This app lists the top 12 'dirtiest' fruits and vegetables that contain the most herbicides and pesticides along with the fifteen cleanest ones. When you go to the grocery store, with a limited budget, you can purchase organic items from the Dirty Dozen and conventionally farmed food from the Clean Fifteen. Because toxins tend to accumulate in fat, I try to buy all my proteins and fats organic. When it comes to cost, I have the same philosophy as I do regarding time. Illness and sickness not only take a tremendous amount of time, but they are extremely costly. I would far sooner invest my time, energy, and money into preventing illness than reacting or responding to it. I consider my groceries and the food I eat an investment in my future.

We also need to recognize that eating a whole foods diet is not boring, tasteless, or deprivational. In fact, it's the total opposite. Eating whole foods is exciting, delicious, satisfying, and, once you get the hang of it, pretty easy. Planning and preparation are key because it does take a little more time to cook and consume whole foods. However, we can revise our thinking around this as well. Instead of looking at it as a hardship, look at it as a labor of love. Cooking with real foods is a wonderful opportunity to fuel your body with life-sustaining nutrients that will ensure robust health and vitality. Whenever I am in the kitchen preparing food, I remind myself how fortunate I am that I can shop for, and cook, these wonderful nourishing ingredients that are going to keep my body healthy for many years to come. It is *not* a hardship, nor do I feel deprived in any way.

Another tenet I like to advocate is 70/30. Realistically, in today's busy world, it's virtually impossible to eat clean, nutrient-dense, organic whole foods 100% of the time. But, the body is an amazing machine and it can function optimally if you give it what it needs 70–80% of the time. The other 20–30% of the time, life happens. We know there are going to be situations when it's difficult to adhere to our whole foods diet and there are going to be times when you just want a treat. On occasion, I have been known to enjoy an ice cream cone on a hot sunny day. If I'm on vacation in Italy, I am eating the pasta. When I go the Calgary Stampede, or any other fair, I must have a corn dog, smothered in mustard. 70/30!

I also don't like to eat until I'm stuffed or feeling uncomfortable. The Japanese have a philosophy called Hara Hachi Bu, it essentially translates to "eat until you are 80% full." It takes

20 minutes for your stomach to send a signal to the brain that it's full. This means you can keep eating for a long time before you even know you're full. I like to eat slowly and mindfully and only eat until I feel luxuriously satisfied. There's no need to stress your digestion by overeating.

I am often asked what I eat on an average day. I think some people believe I sit around eating seaweed and kale all day. My dad included. He used to say that my husband deserved a gold medal for eating the same diet as me. Nothing could be further from the truth. I eat yummy and delicious food every day. I do my best to eat a varied, nutrient-dense diet with a combination of cooked and raw foods. Raw foods are so important to our diet because they are hydrating and they contain enzymes which support digestion and take some pressure off our liver and pancreas. Manufactured food is dead and, hence, devoid of any enzymes. Once we heat food beyond 118°F we also kill off the enzymes. As such, I try and incorporate raw foods in every meal and if I don't get any raw food with my meals, then I try and make sure my snacks are raw. Here are some examples of my typical meals.

Breakfast:

I like to have something nutrient-dense for breakfast, full of fat, fiber, or protein. I find breakfast is a great time to incorporate raw foods. Some of my favorite options include:

- **Chia pudding** – there are various recipes available online.
- **Smoothie** – I always start with a base of spinach or kale and add fruit, almond butter, coconut water, coconut milk, and cinnamon. Variations might be to add raw cacao (full of magnesium, iron, and zinc), hemp hearts, shredded coconut, liquid chlorophyll, a good quality protein powder, etc., it depends on my mood and I what I have in the house.

- **Yogurt parfait** - As you know, I avoid cow dairy. However, I make an exception with plain organic full fat yogurt. Because it's been fermented, it is much easier to digest and the plain version is full of beneficial probiotics. In my yummy parfait, I generally use frozen fruit (this ensures there is some fruit juice) at the bottom of the bowl sprinkled with chia seeds. To this, I add a few dollops of the plain yogurt and mix just until combined. Over this I sprinkle cinnamon and then go crazy with the toppings — cacao nibs, almonds, shredded coconut, and my homemade date-sweetened granola. The sky is the limit and it is delicious no matter what you add! I often throw this breakfast in to a mason jar so I can grab and go if I have a busy morning.
- **Monkey bowl** — I always make this when I have leftover brown rice. On top of the rice, I add some fruit (banana and pear are my favorite), shredded coconut, cacao nibs, cinnamon, nuts, and almond butter. Very similar to the toppings I use for my yogurt parfait.
- **Scrambled or fried eggs**
- **Piece of fruit with nuts**

Lunch:

More often than not, I have a salad for lunch which provides me a good dose of raw. In addition to the greens, I add some other vegetables such as shredded daikon, grated carrots, cucumbers, celery, sprouts, tomatoes, or peppers. I also try to jazz it up by adding other interesting ingredients like avocado, seeds, nuts, coconut chips, orange segments, diced apple, or raisins. I always make my own dressing; the commercial ones are usually full of preservatives, sugar, and other yucky things I want to avoid. Making salad dressing is so easy. I start with organic extra virgin olive oil and then add a vinegar — balsamic and apple cider vinegar are my go-tos. To this I add some garlic, sea salt, pepper, and some other herbs and spices depending on the type of salad. For example, if I make a butter lettuce salad with oranges, avocado, cucumbers, and almonds, I feel like this is a light and fresh salad so I go with olive oil, apple cider vinegar, sea salt, and a little garlic. If it's a heartier salad with romaine lettuce, tomatoes, cucumbers, and peppers, I feel like it needs something more robust so I use olive oil, balsamic vinegar, garlic, dried basil, and salt and pepper. It really is up to you and whatever makes your taste buds happy.

Other awesome lunch options include:

- **Leftovers**.
- **Soup** — I have several quick and easy soup recipes that take no more than 30 minutes to put together.
- **Grain salad** — I will often cook a pot of quinoa, barley, brown rice, or some other whole grain. While the grains are cooking, I will cut up a variety of raw vegetables — carrots, celery, tomatoes, cucumbers, sprouts, pea pods, or purple cabbage and add that to the cooked grains. I add my homemade dressing, and voila! You have a delicious, hearty, and satisfying salad.
- **Veggie burgers** — I have found a few clean, ready-made veggie burgers that I always keep in the freezer for a quick and easy lunch. I pair it with a cucumber salad or some sprouts and I'm good to go.
- **Quinoa and fried eggs** — this is one of my favorites and I have been known to eat this for supper, too! It's quick, easy, and tastes delicious. I like my eggs slightly runny so the yolk soaks into the quinoa... heaven. Another option is to sauté a bunch of veggies (my favorite combination is onion, mushrooms, zucchini, spinach, and tomatoes)

and serve my fried eggs on top of this bed of savory vegetables. It is equally delicious.

- **Sprouted grain toast with mashed avocado and sliced cucumbers** — this is so good and is ready to eat in minutes.

Supper:

I always make an effort to plan my suppers out for the week. That way I am never at a loss for what to make. My sister, one of the busiest people on the planet, orders her meals from a delivery service. Everything she needs to prepare a healthy, whole foods dinner is ready for her when she gets home from work. All she has to do is assemble and prepare the ingredients for a delicious and wonderful dinner that did not require a whole lot of thought to prepare. I think this a great idea for busy people.

On a night where I am tired or pressed for time, I might just have a protein (chicken breasts, turkey sausage, or fish) with three vegetables. I try to have two cooked vegetables and one raw. For example, I might bake some fish and serve that with sautéed Swiss chard, lightly steamed cauliflower, and a fennel celery salad.

If I have more time, I like to prepare a more involved meal such as Turkey Shepherd's Pie with faux mashed potatoes (pureed cauliflower), Chicken Enchiladas, Sweet and Sour Pork stir fry, homemade veggie burgers (thank you Oh She Glows for the best veggie burger *ever*), or red Thai curry. And there are nights when we might order in a pizza, invoking my 70/30 philosophy.

I rarely eat red meat. Let's face it, even the World Health Organization, a mainstream agency, has confirmed red meat is carcinogenic. And, meat is also inflammatory to the body. I eat primarily organic chicken, turkey, and fish as my animal proteins. However, I make a point of going vegetarian two to three days a week. The research really does indicate that a plant-strong diet reduces the risk of all kinds of health problems. In a study called the "Lifestyle Heart Trial," published in 1990, Dr. Dean Ornish was able to scientifically prove that a diet consisting of whole grains, vegetables, legumes, and fruits combined with supplements, stress management, and exercise can reduce, and even reverse, coronary blockages. People are dying of coronary blockages. If people knew they could reverse this health condition through good nutrition and lifestyle changes, it would save lives. The power of diet never ceases to amaze me. And this study was published back in 1990.

Over the last 25 years, the science continues to reinforce the importance of a plant-strong diet for good health. The average North American requires about 30-40 grams of protein/day which is totally achievable even if you don't eat meat. Unfortunately, most of us are getting double that number while only getting about ½ the fiber we require. We are clearly eating too much protein and not enough roughage. John Robbins (of Baskin-Robbins fame) has done a tremendous amount of work trying to educate the general population on the benefits of a plant-strong diet and I find his work most informative. I am not willing to disregard all this research at the risk of my own health. As such, I work hard at ensuring my diet is full of plant-based proteins, along with lots of fruits and vegetables.

Snacks:

Eating a clean, whole foods diet is never about going hungry or depriving yourself. I eat a lot of food in one day and I do not eat low fat and I do not count calories. My philosophy, and it has served me well, is that if you are eating whole foods, you don't have to worry about grams, calories, measurements, servings, or fats. That's the beauty of a whole foods diet. This isn't to say that I stuff my face with anything and everything all day long. It's more about listening closely to the signals your body is sending and nourishing it with wholesome foods. If I'm not hungry, I don't eat. And sometimes, if I'm hungry, I try drinking water to see if it's just dehydration. If I am truly hungry, I will eat and I want my snacks to nourish my body just as much as anything else. Nutrient density is always my goal. Some of my choices include:

- Apple with almond butter & hemp hearts
- Guacamole or hummus with black bean chips
- Hard boiled eggs
- Raw cacao date balls (or some other energy/protein balls)
- Fruit
- Muhummarra dip with veggies (muhummarra is the most amazing dip made with roasted red peppers and walnuts — there are lots of recipes online)
- Homemade popcorn with organic butter
- Homemade Trail mix or a handful of nuts
- Celery with almond butter
- Paleo banana bread (my favorite one is from The Civilized Caveman)

The other day I had some leftover brown rice in the fridge, so a Monkey Bowl was clearly on the menu for my breakfast. I added a sliced banana, raw cacao nibs, cinnamon, coconut chips, a few pecans, and then I drizzled almond butter over everything. Each mouthful was different and delicious! Every bite made me smile and I remember thinking: "There is no way someone could get the same satisfaction, the same pleasure, or the same nutrient density eating a bowl of boring extruded grain cereal like corn flakes". It's just not possible. Revising your diet is not a hardship. It's wonderful and delicious, but, more importantly, it is critical to your long term health and wellness.

● ● ●

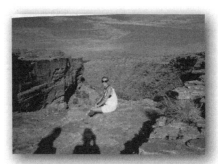

1985 -backpacking through
the Australian outback

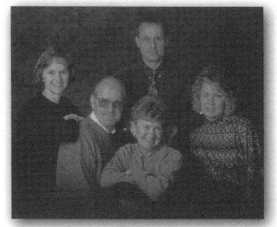

1991 – a family photo; note my "moon
face" (a side effect of the steroids)

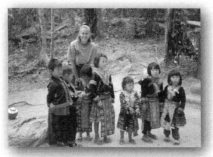

1993 – backpacking
through Thailand

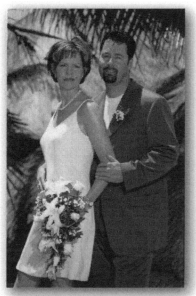

1999 – our wedding in Cancun

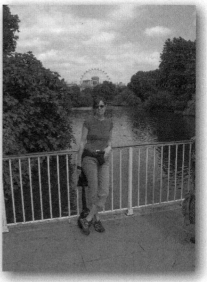

2005 – traveling through Europe;
this photo was taken in London

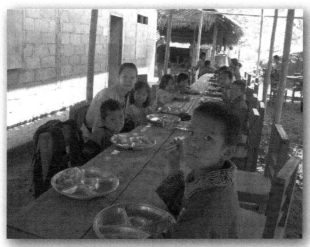

2007 – volunteering in Burma

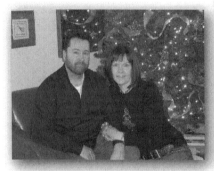

2008 – Ric and me celebrating
Christmas at my sister's

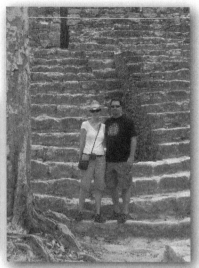

2009 – Ric and me in Coba, Mexico

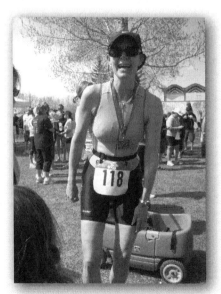

2009 – competing in
my first triathlon

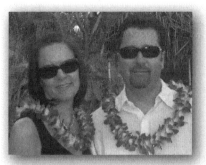

2010 – Ric and me in Hawaii

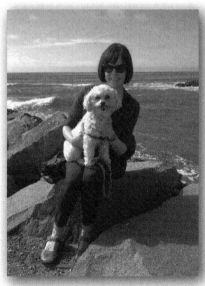

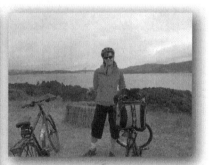

2014 – cycling in San Francisco; this
photo was taken on Angel Island

2014 – me and my pooch,
Jai Jai, enjoying the sun in
southern California

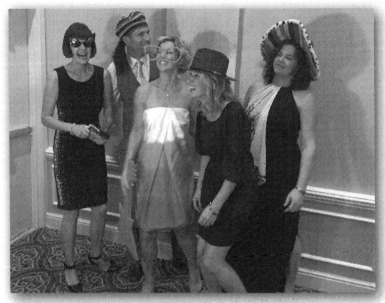

2015 – Canadian School of Natural Nutrition;
graduation celebration with my fellow grads

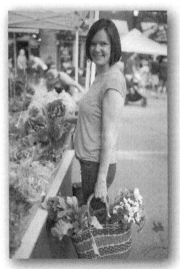

2017 – shopping at a farmer's
market in Edmonton, AB

CHAPTER 9

Step III: Repair the Digestive Tract

Modern medicine is a negation of health. It isn't
organized to serve human health, but only itself, as an
institution. It makes more people sick than it heals
— IVAN ILLICH

I love the metaphor of comparing your health to a garden. Your health is exactly like a garden; you have to sow the seeds, tend to them lovingly, water and weed your garden, and nurture the soil. When something happens to weaken or diminish the garden (i.e., a hail storm, frost, drought, etc.), you have to work extra hard to nurture it back to abundance. Your physical health is no different.

Imagine you have a beautiful, healthy tree growing in your garden. Over time, you notice the tree is unwell, the bark is peeling, and the leaves are turning brown and falling off. You call an expert who specializes in the health of trees. After examining the tree, the expert recommends painting the trunk brown, painting the remaining leaves green, and stapling additional fake leaves onto the branches to fill it out, giving an appearance of health. Do we not agree that is a ridiculous and preposterous approach? If you want a healthy tree, you can't just cover up the problem;

we need to dig deeper into the soil and look at the root system to understand why this tree is failing. And yet, with our own health, we seem to be quite willing to paint the trunk and staple on green leaves in an attempt to look healthy without digging deeper to understand the underlying root cause of our unwellness.

Our traditional approach to health and wellness seeks to reduce symptoms (painting leaves), but does not address root causes. In our current medical system, we have even gone beyond just painting the leaves and we have started cutting off whole branches and replacing them with artificial ones. Sometimes we don't even replace them at all, but just hope that the tree can somehow mend itself despite the missing parts. Can this approach really produce a healthy tree or, more importantly, a healthy body?

In our bodies, the root system of our garden is our gut, otherwise known as the digestive tract. As I mentioned earlier, before chronic illness, there is inflammation and before inflammation, there is gut dysfunction. The truth is, most illnesses today (including conditions that are being diagnosed in epidemic proportions) can be linked back to an unhealthy gut. Over 2,000 years ago, Hippocrates said, "All disease begins in the gut". This still holds true today, but, sadly, nobody seems interested in building health from the inside out — we all want to paint our leaves. In my case, western medicine tried to reduce my inflammation and gastrointestinal symptoms through the use of pharmaceuticals without ever looking deeper. Not one doctor ever suggested I could strengthen or fortify my digestive tract with food. Not one doctor ever questioned what I was eating that might be promoting the disease process. I was continually told that the genesis of autoimmune conditions is a mystery and there was nothing I could have done differently to prevent the development of Crohn's disease. I know now that is a patent untruth.

The importance of good gut health cannot be overstated. It is the cornerstone, the foundation, of our physical health. I believe the majority of people today are living with imbalanced, unhealthy digestive tracts and suffering the consequences to one degree or another. Signs of an unhealthy gut include:

- Acid reflux
- Excess phlegm and mucous
- Gas/bloating
- Skin disorders
- Recurring infections (i.e., tonsillitis, sinusitis, ear infections, etc.)
- Frequents colds/flu
- Allergies
- Mood swings
- Bad breath
- Yeast infections
- Fatigue
- Aches and pains
- Premature aging
- Loose stools or constipation

Most people assume these are completely harmless and benign symptoms that everyone experiences. But, the truth is, these signs of an unhealthy gut can often lead to more chronic and serious conditions. In my case, it was Crohn's disease. I experienced pretty much every symptom on that list, and yet not one doctor *ever* linked them to what I was eating. In our traditional medical approach, these symptoms are often attributed to the unavoidable wear and tear of daily life. They are not recognized as signs of an unhealthy gut or as the underlying cause of illness. The good news is that most of these symptoms can be resolved through some loving attention to the roots and soil of your garden.

The gut (made up of several organs) is referred to as your "second brain" and it performs a myriad of essential functions that affect every single cell in the body, from your bones to your skin and everything in-between. This is why gut dysfunction can manifest in the unlikeliest of body parts. For example, when you notice a rash on your skin you will likely address it with a topical treatment instead of recognizing it as a sign of gut dysfunction. Remember my grand-daughter's eczema cleared up when she changed her diet? When we repair the digestive tract, many of our symptoms will actually resolve and we start to feel significantly better.

The digestive tract includes the mouth, stomach, liver, small intestine, large intestine, pancreas, and gallbladder. All of these organs work in synergy to keep our digestive tract functioning optimally. When one of them is imbalanced, it has a negative impact on the entire system. Repairing the digestive system starts with your choice of food (essentially the fertilizer for your garden); and as I said in steps 1 and 2 (Reduce Inflammation and Revise Your Diet), the body requires *whole* foods; live and good quality foods; foods that are as close to nature as possible.

The reason whole foods are so important is because the food you eat is largely responsible for the type of gut flora you have living in your large intestine. In my mind, good gut bacteria is the single most important component of a healthy digestive tract. There are trillions of bacteria living in your gut; some of them good, some not so good and some are even harmful. Unfortunately, the standard North American diet does a poor job of repopulating the good strains of gut flora and, as such, many people are plagued with bacterial overgrowth including candida.

The emerging research on the importance of gut bacteria is astounding. Poor gut health is being linked to everything from Alzheimer's to obesity, autoimmune disorders, and cancer. Some people are even turning to fecal transplants in an attempt to recolonize their digestive tract with healthy bacteria. Nourishing our inner gut ecology is critical to a healthy body. What you eat every day determines what bacteria live in your gut and whether those bacteria will support vibrant health or lead you down the road to illness and infirmity. Overeating, eating too many processed or refined foods, drinking chlorinated water, smoking, and the overuse of antibiotics tends to promote the growth of pathogens in our digestive tract.

Interestingly enough, steroids (which are often used in the treatment of inflammatory bowel disease) destroy good gut flora. The drug prescribed to help reduce the inflammation associated with Crohn's disease is also setting the stage for more inflammation. What a vicious cycle! I remember when I would try to wean off the steroids, my symptoms would flare up with a vengeance. I now understand that the steroids were wiping out any natural ability I had to control the inflammation, so it's not surprising that my body was unable to find any semblance of health.

Lucky for us, we can replenish the good bacteria in our guts by focusing on fermented foods and supplementing with a good quality probiotic. Fermentation was used for centuries to preserve food before the invention of refrigeration. The process allows bacteria to break down the starches and sugar in food, producing something called lactic acid which is a natural preservative. Fermentation also helps make the nutrients in food more bio-available so it's a double whammy of goodness when you consume fermented foods.

Fermented foods are rich in enzymes and health promoting bacteria (probiotics). Probiotics are anti-microbial. They metabolize cholesterol and they manufacture B vitamins (B3, B5, B6, B12, biotin, folic acid) as well as Vitamin K. They break down toxins, they promote peristalsis, they prevent and decrease inflammation, and they maintain a healthy PH balance in the body. I try and incorporate fermented foods into my diet regularly:

sauerkraut, kefir, kimchi, and miso are all fermented foods I love. You must be careful to ensure you are buying foods that have been traditionally fermented versus mass-produced products that mimic fermentation but don't actually contain any beneficial bacteria. To be clear, any food that has been pasteurized is devoid of probiotics because the pasteurization process kills off all the beneficial bacteria. Many commercially produced yogurt products claim to have probiotics, but this is just not the case. In addition to being pasteurized, these products also contain added sugar, dyes, and perhaps even artificial sweeteners which do not provide an environment in which the bacteria can live.

Along with eating fermented foods, I believe probiotic supplementation is also helpful. I am convinced probiotic supplements saved my life and can help you improve your health. Changing the ecology of your gut is paramount for your overall health and well-being.

When discussing ways to repair the digestive tract, the liver also requires special consideration. The liver is an especially hard-working organ; it is involved in over 200 jobs, so when it gets overburdened, it can wreak havoc in the entire body, including our brain. The liver is the filter for our blood and has the important job of screening for and detoxifying every toxin we absorb, inhale or ingest. Toxins include any alcohol, drug, medication, sugar, coffee, or processed and refined foods laden with pesticides, chemicals, preservatives, and all the other unnatural additives found in our food today. As such, we want to show love to our liver on a daily basis by eating real food. Manufactured food is dead food; it does not nourish our garden and will ultimately contribute to poor gut function. Not only is it full of toxins, it is devoid of all nutrients and enzymes. Enzymes are what support the liver and other digestive organs in digesting and assimilating nutrients. When you eat dead food, the entire digestive tract is stressed because it has to work extra hard to ensure proper digestion — in other words, the food does nothing to help or support the process. Think about stressing the gut meal after meal, day after day, week after week, month after month, year after year for an entire lifetime. The digestive tract cannot continue to function optimally in these circumstances.

Good chewing, simple as it sounds, is also imperative to your overall digestive health. Digestion starts in the mouth and good chewing stimulates a cascade of events that are critical to proper digestion, absorption, elimination, and optimal gut function. The action of chewing triggers our body to start releasing important gastric secretions (HCL, pepsin, bile) that are going to help breakdown our food into molecules that can be easily assimilated and utilized by the body. It also triggers peristalsis which will help the body move food through our digestive tract.

Improper chewing can also lead to a myriad of potential problems. For example, the stomach produces enough hydrochloric acid (HCL) to neutralize pretty much any foodborne pathogen or bacteria that may be present. However, if you have *not* chewed your food properly, the stomach will under produce HCL, leaving you vulnerable to food poisoning and other foodborne illnesses. In addition, pepsin, the enzyme needed to digest protein, is only activated in the presence of HCL. So, if your stomach is not producing sufficient HCL, you are unable to digest protein and this can lead to nutritional deficiencies. In fact, amino acids (the by-product of protein break down) are the building blocks for our immune system; therefore, if you are not digesting proteins properly your immune function will also be compromised. And beware of antacids or prescriptions drugs that suppress your HCL production. Suppressing stomach acid will surely result in health issues.

The other problem if you don't chew your food properly is that the digestive organs (pancreas, gall bladder, intestines) have to work *extra* hard to break down the big chunks of food that were swallowed prior to being masticated into smaller, more manageable sizes. When your body is spending all its time and resources on digestion, it has to forgo other important functions such as immune response, hormone production, purification of the blood, regulation of blood glucose levels, bile production, etc., and this leaves you vulnerable to other health problems. Additionally, large particles of undigested food that the body doesn't recognize as a useable building block (i.e., starch, amino acid, and fatty acid), will be identified as an invader and the body will mount an immune response against that food particle which can lead to allergies, inflammation, leaky gut syndrome, and food sensitivities.

I recommend chewing each mouthful a minimum of 25 times. That may seem like a lot if you are used to eating processed and refined food, but when you make the switch to real food, you will discover it takes more chewing to properly break it down in the mouth. For people with inflammatory bowel disease, digestion is already compromised, so anything you can do to support this process is beneficial and something as simple as good chewing can go a long way towards improving your health and gut function. Even after I had recovered from my Crohn's disease I still struggled with digestion. My digestive tract is full of scar tissue and missing large sections, so my bowel function was always messed up. I would often struggle with extremes; constipation and/or loose stools. I always dreamed of finding a happy medium. When I started chewing my food properly, I was amazed at the changes. I started having regular bowel movements! I had found a pretty consistent, happy medium.

In addition to following the above guidelines for repairing digestive health, there are a number of nutrients that are beneficial to the overall functioning of our gut. These can be used at times when your gut function is compromised (perhaps during a flare-up), but also as a proactive measure to keep the digestive tract healthy and fortified. Some of these can be obtained through diet and others, like digestive enzymes, come from supplementation. A full list of these gut-friendly nutrients can be found in Part III in the chapter entitled Gut Health 101.

● ● ●

CHAPTER 10

Step IV: Rebuild the Immune System

The art of healing comes from nature,
not from the physician.
Therefore the physician must start with
nature, with an open mind
— PARACELSUS

O ur immune system is a complex organization consisting of numerous body parts. Our large intestine has very specific tissue, Mucosa Associated Lymphatic Tissue (MALT), that comprises about 70–80% of our immune system. So, a strong and fortified immune system is the result of good gut health. With inflammatory bowel disease, gut health is essentially nonexistent, ergo our immune system is wiped out! It's a double whammy. The tonsils and appendix are also made up of MALT tissue. Western medicine removes these organs readily without a second thought, but they are important components of our immunity and, if they are malfunctioning, it means your immune system is compromised. The answer is *not* removing them. The answer is rebuilding the immune system.

Everything I recommended in the previous chapters helps to rebuild our immune system. Guidelines such as focusing on a live, natural, good quality whole foods diet; avoiding processed, refined, and chemically laden food; chewing our food well; and eliminating food sensitivities all help support our digestive health which, in turn, strengthens our immune function.

With autoimmune conditions, there is a school of thought that suggests you do not want to boost the immune system as it's your immune system that is supposedly attacking the body in the first place and we don't want to fuel that fire. I do not buy in to this philosophy. I do not believe the body turns on itself. In my opinion, this is a convenient theory, developed by the traditional medical model, to blame the victim and not have to take responsibility for what might be going wrong. My belief is that the body understands, innately, how to support optimal health but, struggles to do so when it does not get the proper nutrients. However, whether you buy into this theory or not, there is overwhelming evidence to suggest that building the immune system is beneficial in *any* circumstance. In this chapter, I will focus on strategies that are good for building and fortifying your immune function (not boosting it) as well as a variety of lifestyle factors that will support your immunity in general.

Once I started down the road of eating a whole foods diet, I stopped getting sick. Even though I often worked in environments where I was surrounded by sick people, I didn't succumb. I always find it funny when people continue to blame their sickness or illness on being exposed to other sick people. Nobody else is making you sick. In some cases, viruses and bacteria can certainly be transferred from one person to another but, if you are one of those people who are plagued with frequent colds and infections, then your immune system is compromised. Period. As I have said before, the body is not made for sickness; it is made for robust health year-round. If you give the body what it needs, it will respond by giving you optimal performance including protection from colds and flus!

There is no doubt that chronic inflammation has a serious negative impact on the immune system and makes us more vulnerable to illness. I also believe that our constant exposure to toxins and chemicals creates a perpetual drain on our immune function. The average North American has up to 600 chemicals circulating in their body and newborns have been found to have upwards of 200. There are studies to suggest that we take in between 8 and 15 pounds of chemicals into our body every year. It is estimated that women can absorb five pounds of chemicals each year from our daily makeup routine alone. On average, women apply 126 different ingredients to their skin daily, and 90% of them have never been evaluated for safety. I was definitely one of these women.

Chemicals like formaldehyde and arsenic are found in many products — some of which I was ingesting or applying on a regular basis. Sodium lauryl sulfate (SLS), a surfactant, detergent, and emulsifier is found in nearly all shampoos, scalp treatments, hair color, toothpastes, body washes and cleansers, make-up foundations, liquid hand soaps, laundry detergents, and bath oils and salts. The manufacturing process for SLS produces dioxane, a carcinogenic by-product. Yuck! It took me years and all kinds of research to figure this out. I had no idea that the products I was using on a daily basis were so damaging to my body. We would never knowingly expose ourselves (or our children) to harmful chemicals with serious side effects. And yet, most people are unknowingly doing this on a daily basis creating added stress on immune function.

Clean water is another important nutrient for your immune system. I think it's likely that a large portion of the population is walking around in a state of dehydration without realizing it. Often times, the first sign of hunger is a really just your body's way of saying I'm dehydrated. Our body is made up of 60% water. Water is needed for every bodily function we have: digestion, elimination and metabolism. Every organ, every tissue, and every cell need water to function properly. Water carries mineral salts and electrolytes to our heart ensuring optimal cardiac function. Water can increase energy levels, improve your skin, flush toxins, promote weight loss, and reduce muscle cramping. We can't dispute the importance of water, but we do need to address quality. All water treatment plants add chlorine to the water, chlorine is toxic and I, for one, do not want to be consuming it. Chlorine kills good gut bacteria, and we can't afford to lose any of our good gut flora. The government of Canada website even acknowledges that chlorine reacts with organic matter naturally found in the water, such as decaying leaves, and forms chemical by-products called trihalomethanes (THM's) which include chloroform. Do we want these chemicals in our bodies creating a constant drain on our immune function? I think not.

Some municipalities even add fluoride to the water. The fluoride added to water, and other commercial goods, is not naturally derived fluoride. It's actually a toxic industrial waste product and is linked to Alzheimer's, thyroid dysfunction, lower cognitive function, and immune dysfunction to name a few. If that's not enough to deter you from drinking tap water, studies all over North America are consistently finding other contaminants in our water such as, lead, radon, mercury, arsenic, pesticides, plastics, disinfectants, radiation, petroleum products, and pharmaceuticals. It's a toxic soup.

I stopped drinking tap water over 20 years ago. I use a reverse osmosis system in my house for all my drinking and cooking water. But, I am also concerned about bathing and showering because you absorb three times more chemicals through your skin than you do by ingesting them. As such, I also have a water softening system that filters the chemicals out of my bath and shower water. It's an extra layer of protection. When I go to my mom's house, I take a pair of rubber gloves to wear while washing dishes so I don't exposure my hands to the unfiltered tap water. You can buy inexpensive filters for your shower head to ensure you don't absorb any nasty chemicals while you are trying to get clean. In an effort to avoid chlorine and fluoride, I have also stopped going into chlorinated pools and hot tubs, I use a fluoride-free toothpaste, and I opt out of fluoride treatments at the dentist. I believe this helps my immune system function more efficiently. We also need to take a look around our environment and consider where we can reduce our chemical exposure. I started using all-natural cleaning products and laundry and dish detergents over 15 years ago; there are a variety of options now available and you can even make your own with water, vinegar, essential oils, baking soda, and a few other common ingredients. There is no need to have toxic chemical cleaning products in your house. It's not good for you, your children, or pets if you have them.

Plastics also emit a variety of chemicals that disrupt our hormones. Storing food in plastic is especially bad because those chemicals can leach out of the plastic into your food. It's virtually impossible to eliminate plastic from your home, but you can certainly reduce your exposure. I have replaced all plastic food containers with glass, my bowls are all glass or stainless steel, my water bottle is glass, and my cutting board is made of recycled wood fiber composite. Instead of using plastic wrap for storing pieces of fruits and vegetables in the fridge, I use a beeswax wrap called Abeego (https://canada.abeego.com/). It's a nice alterative to plastic.

Aluminum is generally recognized as a neurotoxin and is linked to things like Alzheimer's and other brain dysfunction. To be safe, I avoid it whenever possible. I refuse to drink out of an aluminum can and I have replaced aluminum foil with parchment paper in the kitchen. Other sources of aluminum that not everyone knows about include aspirin, antacids, antiperspirants, baking powder, and some commercial oatmeals. Read your labels!

Over the years, I have also worked hard to go completely natural with all my self-care products. Years ago, this was challenging, but nowadays there are a variety of organic options available to us — deodorants, toothpastes, soaps, shampoos, make up, moisturizers, and shampoos to name a few. I always say, if you can't pronounce the ingredients, you probably don't want to put it in *or* on your body. Ask yourself, "Would I eat this?". And, if not, then don't put it on your body. I think one way to clean up your beauty regimen is to simplify your routine and make your own products. Coconut oil can replace a whole slew of products, from skin moisturizers to hair care. EWG's Skin Deep database (http://www.ewg.org/skindeep/) can help you find personal care products that are free of phthalates and other potentially dangerous toxins that stress our immune system.

I make many of my own personal care products. I make a body scrub out of coconut oil, cane sugar, and essential oil. I have made my own deodorant out of coconut oil, arrowroot powder, bentonite clay, and essential oil. I remember I was away for the weekend and, when I went to get ready for bed, I realized I had forgotten my facial wash. Lucky for me, I was able to use my deodorant to wash my face! My nieces are also big on making their own products for their children. They are making diaper creams from beeswax, shea butter and coconut oil as well as, baby powder with arrowroot powder, cornstarch, and some essential oils. It's so easy and you can feel good about using these products because they don't contribute to our toxic load.

We cannot get away from chemicals — we ingest them, we inhale them, and we absorb them through our skin every single day. They wreak havoc in the body; they weaken our immune system, they damage our cells, they speed up aging, they stress our organs of detoxification, they reduce efficiency of all body systems and they produce free radicals.

When I first heard about free radicals, I wrote them off as some weird science thing. I had no clue what they were; they weren't tangible to me in any way and I had no frame of reference in which to understand this theory. However, when I went to the Canadian School of Natural Nutrition, I learned about free radicals and I came to understand how damaging they are to the body!

I am not a scientist, so I will explain the concept of free radicals in the way that makes sense to me. Free radicals are molecules that have lost an electron — it's like a missing body part. Without that electron the molecule becomes unstable. I like to call them "rogue" molecules. They begin to covet their neighbor's electrons and will stop at nothing to get the electron they are missing. They are like terrorists in the body. They attack and damage other molecules indiscriminately, disrupting normal cell activity and leading to a chain reaction of destruction. The damage will depend on which molecules are the victims of the attack. If the cell damage is in our blood vessels, it can lead to a hardening and thickening of the arteries, eventually leading to cardiovascular dysfunction. Free radicals can also cause significant damage to the immune system.

To be clear, our own body produces free radicals as a result of normal metabolism and energy production. But, environmental things like pollution, cigarette smoke, chemicals, synthetic fragrance, pharmaceuticals, and even too much sunlight can also produce free radicals. Inflammation in the body is a major producer of free radicals as well. This is not good news; chronic inflammation = increased free radicals in the body. It's a vicious cycle. Lucky for us, there is an antidote for free radicals and they are called antioxidants. When antioxidants come into contact with a free radical, they willingly and freely give up one of their electrons to complete the free radical and stop the carnage and destruction. Even though the antioxidant gives up an electron, they are able to stay neutral and not cause further damage. A healthy body produces several powerful antioxidants such as, glutathione, lipoic acid, and superoxide dismutase, but, we can also get some amazing backup antioxidants through our dietary intake. Vitamins A, C, E, and the mineral selenium are all amazing antioxidants and should be consumed, in large quantities, on a daily basis.

Aside from antioxidants there are some other super powerful nutrients that can enhance and support immune function such as Vitamin D, magnesium, garlic and zinc. The benefits of these vitamins and minerals are legion and much too lengthy to list in detail here. Chapter 13, The Secret to Immunity, provides more in-depth information related to specific nutrients and how they can fortify the body. I think it helps to understand why certain things are important to your health as this may increase your motivation to incorporate them into your day to day life.

The nutrients I have mentioned here and in Chapter 13, are designed to build and fortify the immune system. The immune boosters that I referred to earlier do not build new immune cells; what they do is stimulate and arouse our own immune cells and system so they can respond more efficiently to an invader. As I mentioned, with autoimmune conditions it is traditionally thought the immune system is attacking itself and, therefore, we would not want to stimulate the system which is supposedly attacking us. Supplements such as Echinacea, andrographis, and goldenseal are considered immune boosters and I use all of these on a regular basis. However, given the prevailing theory on auto-immune condition, it's important to use good judgment when considering the use of these supplements.

In terms of lifestyle, there are a variety of recommendations that can further support and enhance your immune system. We have already discussed toxic load, the importance of antioxidants, and the information from the chapters on Reducing Inflammation, Revising your Diet, and Repairing the Digestive Tract is all relevant to building immune function. Other lifestyle tips to keep your immune system strong include getting enough sleep and exercise, lymphatic massage and drainage, managing your stress, earthing or grounding, and practicing good hand washing.

I follow all of the guidelines in this chapter and my immune system has served me very well over the last 20 years. I rarely get sick. In fact, in the last 15 years, I have only been really sick (where I was in bed) on two occasions. This does not mean that

I never feel unwell, but, generally, when I start to feel like I am coming down with something, I can stop it before it gets started. The first thing I do when I start to feel sick is increase my dose of Vitamin C, probiotics, vitamin D, and cod liver oil. I also start drinking green juice — there is nothing that provides a more powerful infusion of nutrients, directly into the body, than vegetable juice. It's amazing! I try not to eat a lot of food because I want my body focused on immune response instead of digesting a bunch of food. Digestion takes a tremendous amount of energy and I need all my resources working on fighting off the invaders. I also use essential oils, both topically and orally. Topically, I massage the oil into acupressure points connected to my lungs, sinuses, throat, and large intestine. I like to use frankincense or Thieves (a blend of Clove, Lemon, Cinnamon, Eucalyptus and Rosemary). If I feel like I have some sinus congestion or a sore throat, I will rub the oil right onto the skin of my throat or over my sinuses. I also add a few drops of the oil to a hot herbal tea (usually turmeric if I am not feeling well) and sip on that throughout the day. Baths in Epsom salts are a must if I'm feeling like my body is under attack; it's detoxifying, it gives me a boost of magnesium, and heat helps kick the immune system into high gear. Plus, it feels so good. I usually add essential oil to the bath as well. If your sinuses are congested, you could try some essential oil of eucalyptus or cedar in the bath to help clear them.

Rebuilding the immune system after it has been ravaged by inflammatory bowel disease is so important and it will benefit you in so many different ways. The body wants to perform optimally and it knows intuitively how to do this. It's just waiting for you to start making some changes so it can support you with vibrant and robust health.

● ● ●

CHAPTER 11

Step V: Reprogram your Thinking

Your body hears everything your mind thinks
— *NAOMI JUDD*

When I went to the Canadian School of Natural Nutrition, there was a significant focus on the interconnection between the mind, body, and spirit. This was a bit of a revelation to me. My mind and spirit were connected to my physical health? It was an "A-ha!" moment. Like most people, I paid lip service to the idea of being positive, thinking positive, and being grateful for what I had. I understood, intuitively, that focusing on the negatives doesn't solve problems, that being critical and judgmental of people around me isn't nice, and that you do unto others as you would have them do to you. Most people understand these concepts, *but* embodying them and living them is a different thing altogether. As part of our course work, we had to read, and write a book report on, a spiritual book. After much research, I found a book called *You Can Heal Your Life* by Louise Hay. I chose it because it was pretty short, so I thought it would be an easy read. Little did I know this book would change my life forever.

You Can Heal Your Life resonated deeply for me and it helped me start to connect the dots of my own recovery from Crohn's. When I started reading the book, I was fascinated by this idea of how thoughts and beliefs can create our reality. This idea of where attention goes, energy flows or the point of power is always in the present moment. Many of us spend so much time reliving our history or obsessing about the future but, we never claim the power that is present in each moment. One thing Louise would often say in the book was that "a thought is just a thought and a thought can be changed." It is such a simple statement, but it carries unbelievable power because it really puts the onus back on us to be responsible for our own well-being. Louise wrote that every thought we think is creating our future and that we create every illness in our body. In fact, Louise had been diagnosed with vaginal cancer in her 50's and within six months was able to rid her body of the cancer through natural and alternative therapies. This was really heady stuff for me. While I had already achieved some pretty amazing physical results in my health, I came to understand I could improve upon that even more by changing how I thought about the world around me.

The book really underlined how much influence I had and that by making some adjustments to how I interpreted things it could have a powerful impact in all areas of my life. I was so intrigued by the concepts I was introduced to in the *You Can Heal Your Life* book, I traveled to San Diego in October 2015 and became a Certified Teacher of Louise Hay's You Can Heal Your Life philosophy. I wanted to be able to bring these concepts to my clients. I was starting to see that you could not have total wellness if you were neglecting a component of the mind, body, and spirit trilogy. I came to realize that you could have wonderful physical health, but if you were feeding your brain a bunch of negativity and limiting thoughts and beliefs, you would not be able to maintain your health. And, by the same token, you could be the most positive thinking person in the world, full of love and forgiveness, but if you were feeding your body a bunch of crap and garbage, you would never achieve vibrant health. In my mind, the two went hand-in-hand.

Dr. Bill Pettit (psychiatrist) has done a tremendous amount of research into the power of thoughts and beliefs and his work suggests that just 30 minutes of negative thinking is enough to start turning off certain genetic switches in our bodies, thus altering our DNA. This is unbelievable power and totally within our control. It's an incredible tool that we can use to our advantage on a daily basis. Think about how we have been conditioned to view illness; we "fight" and wage "war" on diseases but our body is not a battleground and illness is simply the way the body communicates. Unfortunately, this is not the prevailing message we are being given by society.

As I became more aware of how my beliefs could impact my wellness, I started reprogramming all my thoughts to focus more on the positives and I started to seriously question everything I thought I believed. Every time I caught myself thinking something negative or being judgmental about something or someone, I would query where that belief came from and whether it was grounded in truth or just something I was repeatedly told as I was growing up. If I came to realize that a particular belief was not actually serving me I would replace it with something more useful. I introduced a daily devotion exercise where I would express gratitude for everything I had in life versus what I didn't have. I started using positive affirmations to focus on the things that I wanted in my life so I could attract them. Louise was a big proponent of positive affirmations and she suggested that every negative thought you have can be transformed in to a positive one. For example, if your belief is "I never have enough money" then you would start affirming "money comes to me easily and effortlessly." As I mentioned, if energy flows to what you think about, then thinking negative thoughts will only serve to perpetuate more negativity and scarcity in your life. It really is about reprogramming your brain and evaluating what you "think" is true for you. None of us have all the answers so, it behooves each of us to be open and receptive to new ways of viewing the world around us. Based on these new practices, I noticed a profound change in my life. I was happier, the people close to me were happier, and I had a whole new outlook. I felt more powerful than I ever had before. I was more confident about my ability to direct things in a way that would serve my greater good and help me maintain my physical and mental health for years to come. This new way of being reminded me of a quote I had read years ago by Albert Einstein, "We cannot solve our problems with the same thinking we used when we created them". How very accurate but, I think we get caught up in believing our thoughts are actually facts and we struggle to be open and receptive to alternate ways of thinking. I was so grateful to realize I *had* been able to change my thinking in order to get well.

When I started to reprogram my thoughts and beliefs, I had already achieved a solid level of health. So, if you are currently unwell, reprogramming your thoughts will look a little different. You want to start by focusing your attention on wellness, not sickness. Even though you may not feel great, it's important to start talking and thinking as if you are well. And you also want to start talking and thinking in the present. For example, you want to say things like "my body is whole and healthy" rather than "I want to be whole and healthy." This way of framing things is a powerful message for your subconscious mind and helps train your brain to start seeing yourself as better. Pain is registered in the emotional part of the brain so it is *very* important to practice *feeling* and *believing* you are well to help develop new neural pathways.

If you recall from my story, I woke up one morning, really sick, and I intuitively knew there had to be another way of living. That morning was a turning point in my life; I reclaimed my power. Even then, I somehow understood that I had the ability to elicit change in my life. And, after implementing some of the tenets of Louise Hay, I came to appreciate this power more and more. Even before my introduction to Louise, and more strongly afterwards, I believed that health was a choice. Or, perhaps more accurately, health is a series of choices that we make every day. Remember that our thoughts will dictate what kinds of choices we make. We experience life one thought at a time. A thought goes into our limbic system and reverberates around for a while, eventually becoming a belief. Do we believe we are healthy? Do we believe we have power or do we believe that life just happens to us and we have no control? What we think will ultimately determine our reality.

One choice does not make us sick, but numerous unhealthy choices day after day, week after week, month after month *does* make us sick. So, if we start making healthy choices day after day, week after week, month after month, then there is no reason we can't get better. I heard Dr. Bruce Lipton say that only 5% of illness is determined by genetics; the other 95% is a result of lifestyle; diet, exercise and what we believe and think. That means our choices are *powerful* and we do have the ability to achieve vibrant and robust health based on decisions we make every day!

Consider this scenario, a woman gets acid reflux after most meals. She sees her doctor, and to 'treat' this problem the doctor prescribes an antacid (proton pump inhibitor). The antacid suppresses stomach acid which the body needs for proper absorption and assimilation of nutrients, and for good protein digestion. Without good absorption and protein digestion, many of our body systems, including our immune function, become compromised. Subsequently, the woman starts to get headaches (which may or may not be a side effect of the antacid). To 'treat' the headache, she starts taking an OTC pain reliever which further irritates her stomach. Several years later, she develops an ulcer for which she takes another medication and eventually has surgery to remove the ulcer. Meanwhile, she continues taking antacids and eating the same as always. Shortly thereafter, she develops high blood pressure (which is linked to the use of antacids and other such medications) and so begins taking hypertensive medication. The side effects of this medication include headaches, dizziness, drowsiness, diarrhea, and weight gain. The woman also develops numerous musculoskeletal issues such as joint pain and muscle cramping, which are linked to the fact that her body is not able to absorb certain nutrients — a side effect of her antacid. As her physical health declines, her emotional and mental health worsen because of all her symptoms, so she starts taking anti-depressants. Eventually she has a heart attack and undergoes an operation to repair a heart valve. During recovery, she uses painkillers, antibiotics, and other medications that further deplete the body's natural resources. A few years later, she finds herself diagnosed with an aggressive and debilitating autoimmune condition such as multiple sclerosis or rheumatoid arthritis, and she wonders what could have gone wrong. Her health has deteriorated so sufficiently that she is no longer able to work.

Unfortunately, I don't think this scenario is all that unusual. In fact, it has strong parallels to my own personal story. But, let's backtrack and see how different choices may produce a different result. In this scenario, let's start with the assumption that we believe in our power and our own ability to maintain health; that *all* symptoms are a warning sign from the body; and that the body can innately repair itself if we give it what it needs. A woman gets acid reflux after most meals. The woman starts to pay attention to what she is eating to see if she can make a connection between food and the burning sensation she feels after eating. She starts to eliminate common inflammatory and allergenic foods and pinpoints her stomach discomfort to dairy, gluten and fast food. Along with eliminating these foods from her diet, she starts to supplement with probiotics and digestive enzymes and the acid reflux disappears. As she does not have to take an antacid, she is able to properly digest and assimilate nutrients so the rest of her body stays healthy; she is also able to continue digesting protein properly so her immune system stays strong. When the woman gets a headache, instead of masking it with medication, she continues to look for an underlying root cause. After much investigation, perhaps she links it to biomechanical dysfunction and starts seeing a chiropractor or massage therapist to address her musculoskeletal imbalance. Perhaps she connects it to the MSG in her packaged or processed food, so she cuts that out of her diet. Or perhaps she links it to a mild state of dehydration, so she starts drinking more water consistently throughout her day. Now she has eliminated her stomach distress and her headaches. She is not taking any pharmaceuticals and is therefore not experiencing any side effects. Her stomach is relaxed, her immune system is balanced, and the likelihood of an ulcer and high blood pressure is greatly diminished. Because she has eliminated the foods that she is sensitive to, and is eating more whole foods instead of processed and refined foods, her risk of heart attack is also reduced. Because she feels good, she behaves differently and does not become depressed. Her proactive and holistic approach will help ensure she lives well into old age and dies peacefully in her sleep.

Which scenario do you prefer? The body is an amazing and powerful instrument. It can restore balance and overcome significant infirmity as long as you provide it with the tools it needs to function optimally. I believe it all comes down to what we believe and the choices we make based on those beliefs.

In order to make good choices, we need education. Education is power, but the world of diet and nutrition is confusing. There are so many conflicting views and contradictory recommendations. Is coconut oil good or is it going to cause a heart attack? Will saturated fats make me fat? Should I avoid fruit if I am watching my blood sugar levels? How does one navigate through all the misinformation? We need to have some trustworthy sources. Sources who do not have a vested interest in keeping us sick; we need sources who are actually interested in the truth!

What I find fascinating about much of the health information available to us is that it comes from sources who stand to profit from our choices. It's generally the multinational corporations who manufacture our food and pharmaceuticals that are making all the recommendations. How can we trust these people to tell us what we need when they stand to profit from our unwellness?

These agencies are far more interested in profits than in helping us lead vibrant, robust, and healthy lives. I think trusting these companies to tell us what is in our best interests is akin to trusting the tobacco companies to tell us whether smoking is safe. Unfortunately, they have the loudest and most prominent voices, but that doesn't make them right. We must challenge the way we view this information and start questioning it instead of accepting it blindly. Remember, a thought enters our mind, reverberates around for a while, and eventually becomes a belief. When we repeatedly hear the claims of these multinational companies, with no regular information to challenge it, we start to believe their claims as truth. But, this does not have to be the case. We can reprogram our thoughts to develop new beliefs that will serve our greater good.

There are hundreds of thousands of people, all around the world, who are overcoming serious life-threatening illnesses, including cancer, naturally. What is the difference between them and the people who are sick and pumping their bodies full of chemicals in an attempt to feel good? As I mentioned, I believe it comes down to your beliefs about health and about choice. If you do not feel empowered then you will not seek out options. If you do not believe you have control, then you will follow whatever advice you are given. If you believe that doctors are the experts and you do not have any knowledge about your body, then you will give away your power. If you don't believe you have the ability to make the best decisions for yourself, then you won't ask questions. And, if you believe you are sick and there is nothing you can do, then you will remain sick. Doctors are only human. They are not magical. They do not have all the answers. And, they do *not* always know what is in your best interests. Yet, we seem to be quite willing to entrust our lives to these people. Hippocrates said, "let food be thy medicine" and Thomas Edison said, "the doctor of the future will give no medicine but will interest his patients in the care of the human frame, in diet and in the cause and prevention of disease". I believe 100% in these quotes but do you know how much nutritional training medical doctors receive in school? None. Medical schools do not teach about diet and nutrition even though there is a plethora of research out there confirming diet is one of the most powerful tools in our health arsenal. My own story is a prime example of how food can transform the body.

If you want to get better, you must reclaim your power by reprogramming your thinking. Dr. Bruce Lipton said: "don't believe everything you think". This is great advice! It's time to start challenging your beliefs about health. Start asking questions, start searching out answers, and start educating yourself on how you can improve your wellbeing. Two of my favorite online resources are Dr. Mercola (mercola.com) and Dr. Josh Axe (draxe.com). Dr. Mercola's information is well sourced and researched. If he is posting information on his website, you can be assured it's accurate *and* it's truthful. Dr. Mercola has made it his life's work to expose the litany of lies and misinformation we are being told about health. Make sure you are gathering as much information as you can from reputable sources so you can make informed decisions based on your new beliefs. Your life depends on it.

● ● ●

Part III — Food For Thought

CHAPTER 12
Gut Health 101

A healthy outside starts from the inside
— *ROBERT URICH*

A s you know, I believe gut health is the cornerstone of wellbeing. It's the foundation that allows us to thrive and flourish. Because I spent many years with an unhealthy gut, I take special precautions every day to ensure my gut stays strong and fortified. I have already explained everything I did to repair my digestive tract, but I also wanted to provide you the names of supplements and nutrients that I continue to use on a regular basis. The following list is by no means exhaustive, but these are the nutrients that have helped me keep my digestive system in tiptop shape.

Digestive Enzymes:
Enzymes support digestion, reduce the load on the liver, and ensure that there is less undigested food in the body. Enzymes will also help to alleviate allergies as properly digested food is rendered non-allergenic. In addition, enzymes are anti-inflammatory and have been shown to digest micro-organisms, including candida albicans, toxins, bacteria, and other parasites. Digestive enzymes

can be taken with meals and in between meals. In-between meals, the body uses the enzymes to support the work of metabolic enzymes which are needed for immune support. For people with any type of gut dysfunction, I would highly recommend digestive enzymes. When I am going out and I know I will be eating a big meal or eating foods that may not be easy to digest, I always take a digestive enzyme to support my body. If you don't want to purchase digestive enzymes, you could always substitute 1 tbsp. of apple cider vinegar in a glass of water 30 minutes before eating — this will stimulate HCL production and aid digestion.

Bone Broths:

There has been a lot of hype recently about the health benefits of bone broth. It's all true! Bone broth is an excellent source of amino acids, primarily arginine, glycine, and proline. Not only do these amino acids nourish the gut but, they have numerous other benefits for the body. Glycine plays a role in detoxification, it supports the nervous system, and is used in the synthesis of hemoglobin and bile. Glycine also enhances digestion, supports gut health and helps regulate blood sugar. Proline, especially when paired with vitamin C, supports good skin health. Arginine is known to improve circulation and is beneficial for the health of our blood vessels. Bone broths are also rich in gelatin which is a critical nutrient for optimal digestive health and we should all be striving to improve our digestion.

Commercial bones broths are becoming more and more readily available, but it's really easy and more economical to make at home. I use organic bones (always use organic) and I put it in the slow cooker outside, even in the winter, so the house doesn't smell like a soup factory. I use my bone broths in a variety of ways; I use it as a base for soups or stews, but I also like to drink it on its own with a little salt and butter (the melted butter in the broth adds a rich, salty flavor that I love). I also like to make a chocolate mushroom elixir using beef broth. Bone broth on its own is quite neutral tasting, so it can take on a number of flavors depending what you add. For my mushroom elixir, I take a mushroom powder (these are readily available in any health food store), I happen to like chaga, lion's mane, and reishi, and I add bone broth, a nondairy milk, raw cacao, a dash of pure maple syrup, and a pinch of cayenne pepper. I blend it up and, voila, I have a frothy, chocolatey shake. It is simply delicious and tastes super decadent, but it's chock full of nutrient-dense goodness that does my body good.

Butyric Acid:

Butyric Acid is a short chain fatty acid, which means the body can readily absorb and utilize it. In addition, it repairs gut mucosa. It has a remarkable effect on intestinal permeability and helps restore the integrity of the gut lining. It's also anti-inflammatory. A healthy gut, a gut that is full of beneficial probiotics, produces butyric acid; but, if your large intestine is compromised, you may not be making any of this beneficial nutrient. The other richest source of butyric acid is organic butter from grass-fed cows. Organic butter is a staple in my house. I use it for cooking, baking, over my steamed veggies, on my brown rice, and in my bone broth!

Chlorophyll:

Chlorophyll is anti-microbial and a super potent anti-oxidant to fight free radicals. It supports apoptosis (natural cell death), it's hormone balancing, and enhances immune function. Chlorophyll also promotes healthy digestion by maintaining intestinal flora, detoxifying the body and stimulating bowel movements. It is effective for constipation and can alleviate the discomfort caused by gas. The best food sources are dark green veggies like spinach, kale, Swiss chard, collard greens and broccoli. I like to add a little shot of liquid chlorophyll to my smoothies or water for a little infusion of this health-promoting nutrient.

Fermented foods and probiotics:

I know I have said this before but, probiotics are the basis for good gut health and I believe they were largely responsible for saving my life. I started supplementation of probiotics over 20 year ago and I still take them to this day. They perform a variety of life-sustaining jobs and they are also a boon to immune function, because, as we know, 80% of our immune system lives in our gut. Great food sources include water kefir, sauerkraut, kimchi, plain organic yogurt, tempeh, and miso. Studies show that sauerkraut also stimulates HCL production which we know is critical to digestion. Need I say more? I believe everyone, regardless of age, health, or diet should be eating fermented foods on a regular basis as well as, taking a probiotic supplement. In my family, everyone from my infant grandchildren to my elderly mother take a probiotic supplement and they have all experienced positive benefits as a result.

● ● ●

CHAPTER 13

The Secret to Immunity

You are what you eat, so don't be
fast, cheap, easy or fake
—*UNKNOWN*

I n Step IV, Rebuild the Immune System, I talked about free radicals and how these can stress our immune function. The good news is that there are antidotes for free radicals and they come in the form of antioxidants. The following information will provide you with some insight into why antioxidants are so critical to our overall health and well-being and how you can incorporate more of them into your daily diet to strengthen your immune function.

Vitamin C is a powerful antioxidant. A healthy body requires 500 mg of Vitamin C per hour to function; a body fighting off a virus will use up to 1000 mg/hour. So, feel free to increase your intake of Vitamin C-rich foods during the cold and flu season. Vitamin C supports adrenal function and protects against free radical damage. Vitamin C also helps displace mercury in the body. In addition to supporting immune function, Vitamin C is critical to wound healing. I sustained several deep lacerations in my leg as a result of a bicycling accident a few years ago. I probably should have received stitches but, we were on vacation in San Francisco at the time and, I just assumed I could heal naturally. The wounds eventually became infected and I was prescribed anti-biotics but, I was unwilling to take them unless my life was in jeopardy. I bumped up my intake of Vitamin C and probiotics and, within a few days, the infection was gone but, what was even more amazing is how the skin just seemed to miraculously regenerate and heal. My niece recently had twins and she said vitamin C was critical to her healing after giving birth vaginally. She belongs to a group of other mothers, who also gave birth to twins, and they were all struggling with infections and an inability to heal following their deliveries. My niece healed completely within days of giving birth. Her secret? Mega doses of Vitamin C. There is no denying the amazing ways in which Vitamin C benefits the body. A great way to get your vitamin C is by eating kiwis. Kiwis have the highest amounts of vitamin C than any other food source. Other foods high in vitamin C include citrus fruits, bell peppers, broccoli, Brussel sprouts, butternut squash, papaya, sweet potatoes, and tomatoes.

Increasing your intake of vitamin A, another antioxidant, is also good for immune health. In fact, it stimulates the production of T-cells which are a critical component of our immune system. Vitamin A is important for good vision, it supports skin health and cell growth, and it helps reduce inflammation in the body. Vitamin A comes in two forms: active vitamin A (preformed), also known as retinol, which comes from animal sources, and beta-carotene (a nutrient that can be converted into retinol in the body) which is obtained from plant sources. Active vitamin A is most abundant in fish liver oils (think cod liver oil) along with liver, raw milk, organic yogurt, eggs, and butter. You can also consume beta-carotene and let your body convert it into active Vitamin A. However, if you have diabetes or an underactive thyroid, your ability to make this conversion is compromised. As such, you may want to consider supplementation if you have one of these conditions. Great sources of beta-carotene are carrots, squash, apricots, papaya, sweet potatoes, spinach, and parsley.

Lots of yummy options to get your vitamin A! It's also important to remember that Vitamin A works synergistically with zinc and Vitamin E (so be sure you are getting plenty of those nutrients as well). A deficiency of vitamin A is often easy to detect; little bumps/irritations on the skin, at the back of your upper arm, is a sure indicator you are lacking in this nutrient.

Vitamin E does not get enough recognition. It's super important to the production of sex hormones and it is believed to be heart protective. It's also a powerful antioxidant. Absorption of vitamin E requires pancreatic secretions and bile, so if you have diabetes or your gall bladder has been removed, you may want to consider supplementation. Options to enhance your intake of vitamin E include wheat germ, broccoli, brussel sprouts, whole grains, oatmeal, and eggs.

It's not well-known, but selenium packs a powerful antioxidant punch! It works synergistically with Vitamin E. Selenium has many roles including helping to normalize blood pressure, maintaining healthy hair, and supporting the reproductive system. Selenium also helps counteract the negative effects of mercury in the body. We obtain selenium from garlic, onions, broccoli, and whole grains. Brazil nuts also have high levels of selenium and just three brazil nuts per day will give you what you need. I happen to love brazil nuts, so I know I am getting a good dose of selenium almost daily.

You may have noticed that many of these nutrients work synergistically with each other. This means they require other vitamins, minerals, and co-factors to be optimally utilized by the body. That's why it's *so* important to get as many nutrients as possible from whole foods. Nature ensures that every food we eat has the perfect ratio of vitamins and minerals to ensure the best possible result for our body.

When it comes to immune function, I think there are other nutrients that require special mention. These include garlic, zinc, magnesium, vitamin D and sufficient protein.

Garlic is a potent antibacterial, antiviral, and anti-fungal agent. Garlic also stimulates glutathione production in the body (as mentioned earlier, glutathione is a powerful antioxidant and important liver detoxifier). Ideally it should be consumed raw, and crushed just before eating. When you are starting to feel under the weather, it is a perfect time to crush a clove or two (mix with a little scoop of raw honey if you must) and swallow it down. It's also great to throw it into salad dressings for extra immune support.

Earlier, I mentioned that Vitamin A works synergistically with zinc, another important nutrient for immune system building. Zinc has a number of important roles in the body, including supporting production of HCL in the stomach — and we know how important HCL production is for the body. Zinc also enhances immune function by increasing T-cell production (T-cells are an important component of your immune system). Zinc has also been found to greatly reduce the severity of symptoms from the common cold or flu. For the men in your life, zinc is critical. The highest concentration of zinc in the body is found in the prostate gland, so make sure all the men you know are getting enough zinc in their diets. I happen to love all the foods that are rich in zinc: eggs, pumpkin seeds, sunflower seeds, mushrooms, and seafood. I sprinkle sunflower or pumpkin seeds on *all* my salads. It's nutritious and it adds a nice crunch.

Magnesium is known as nature's tranquilizer. It's such a critical nutrient in the body, and yet most of us are deficient in this mineral. It's easily flushed out of our system by anything that has a diuretic effect such as, caffeine and alcohol. If you are a coffee drinker or enjoy a glass of wine every night, you are likely deficient in magnesium. Magnesium is a co-factor in hundreds of metabolic reactions in the body. According to Dr. Amy Myers, a magnesium deficiency is linked to autoimmune conditions. She writes that "magnesium deficiency has been shown to cause an increased production of pro-inflammatory cytokines, which raise your overall level of inflammation in the body" and we now know that inflammation is generally underlying most illnesses. If a magnesium deficiency promotes inflammation, we want to avoid that at all costs so bring on the magnesium! One of my favorite ways to get an infusion of magnesium is by taking an Epsom salt bath (Epsom salts are magnesium sulfate). Leafy greens and other fresh vegetables are also jam packed with magnesium. Liquid chlorophyll, which is highlighted in chapter 12, is essentially magnesium so you can add a few drops of this to a smoothie or a glass of water to get an extra dose. The market has also been flooded with a variety of new magnesium gels and lotions that can be applied topically. With all these options, there is *no* excuse for a magnesium deficiency.

As an aside, my pooch, Jai Jai, is a shih tzu/poodle mix. Poodles are prone to tears which are brownish red in color due to a pigment called porphyrins. The tears can stain the hair on their face quite dramatically. When Jai Jai was about 5 we started to notice an increase in his tears and staining on his fur following a stay at our house in Southern California. Most products for this problem contain anti-biotics which I was not willing to use. Our holistic vet suggested we start supplementing him with a few drops of liquid chlorophyll in his food on a daily basis, and the tears cleared right up! No more discharge, no more tears, no more staining. So, don't forget about your pets! Their health also benefits from some of the same things I am recommending.

The benefits of vitamin D have been well documented and I think, by now, we all know we should be supplementing with vitamin D. It is important to note there are two types of Vitamin D: Vitamin D2 (ergocalciferol) and D3 (cholecalciferol). I don't want to bore you with an explanation about the differences between the two, but D3 is the one you want to be using. All nutrients are typically processed through the liver and the liver prefers Vitamin D3 as it is more readily metabolized and bio-available to the body.

While we are aware of the need for vitamin D in supporting good bone health, what we often don't realize is that it also plays a significant part in immune function. According to Dr. Mercola, Vitamin D3 has a crucial role in disease prevention and maintaining optimal health. He also writes that Vitamin D can "slash your cancer risk by up to 60% and help reduce the risk of other conditions as well, including type 2 diabetes, chronic inflammation, age-related macular degeneration (the leading cause of blindness), and Alzheimer's disease". If that's not a ringing endorsement for Vitamin D3 supplementation, I don't know what is. The other alternative is to spend time in the sunshine so you can manufacture your own Vitamin D. Unfortunately, we have been programmed to think that we need to slather on the sunscreen before we venture out in to the sunlight. Once again, Dr. Mercola has some very enlightening information on the subject of sun exposure and I think it bears repeating. The below excerpt is copied directly from his website (mercola.com):

"I strongly recommend ample sunlight exposure as your main source of vitamin D, as the sun provides beneficial UVB wavelengths that are needed to optimize your levels.

Although most dermatologists will tell you to avoid the sun to prevent diseases like cancer, exposure can actually aid in skin cancer prevention — and there are studies confirming this. Melanoma occurrence is found to decrease with greater exposure to direct sunlight. According to a study published in the *European Journal of Cancer,* melanoma was found to be more common in workers who spent time indoors, and in body parts that are not exposed to the sun.

The sun emits two types of wavelengths at different periods in a day: UVA rays and UVB rays. Your body requires UVB for vitamin D production. UVA rays, on the other hand, have longer wavelengths and can penetrate the ozone layer, as well as clouds and pollution. Frequent exposure to this type of wavelength increases your risk of skin cancer and photoaging. Occasional exposure of your hands and face to the sun does not constitute appropriate sunlight exposure. To optimize your levels, large portions of your skin needs to be exposed to the sun. However, over exposure to the sun can result in sunburn, which will increase your risk for skin cancer and premature skin aging."

Once you get the proper amount of sunlight, your body will stop producing vitamin D because of its self-regulating mechanism. Here are other important factors in safe sunlight exposure:

1. **Time** — The best time to expose yourself to the sun is as near to solar noon as possible (during Daylight Saving Time, solar noon is typically around 1 pm). UVB rays, unlike UVA rays that are present all throughout the day, are very low in the morning and evening, and are abundant during midday — around 10:00 am to 2:00 pm. Expose yourself to direct sunlight between these times for a short period, and you will have produced the most vitamin D3.

2. **Skin pigmentation** — Fair-skinned people can potentially max out their vitamin D production in just 10 to 20 minutes, or when their skin has turned the lightest shade of pink. However, if you have darker skin, you likely need to remain in the sun longer.

3. **Sensitive body parts** — The skin located around your eyes is thinner compared to other areas on your body. Since it has a small surface area, it will not do much to contribute to vitamin D production. You need to protect this part of your face, as it is very prone to photoaging and premature

wrinkling. I recommend using a safe sunblock or wearing a cap that will keep your eyes in the shade. If you get sunburned, aloe vera is one of the best remedies to help repair your skin. This plant is loaded with powerful glyconutrients that will induce healing. I suggest deriving the gel from a fresh plant.

4. **Using soap** — When UVB rays strike the surface of your skin, your skin will then convert a cholesterol derivative, which will turn into vitamin D3. However, the produced vitamin D3 does not immediately enter your bloodstream. It may take up to 48 hours before the vitamin D3 penetrates into your bloodstream. When you shower immediately after sun exposure, you risk washing away the vitamin D3 formed by your skin and potentially reduce the benefits of sun exposure."

The other important nutrient for building the immune system is protein. When ingested, protein is broken down into constituents called amino acids. Remember that HCL is required in order for protein to be broken down into amino acids and insufficient HCL will result in a protein deficiency. So, part of a healthy immune system is good chewing as this produces more HCL (you had no idea how important it is to chew!). Amino acids are the building blocks of your immune system. All of our white blood cells and tissues of the immune system require protein. There are also specific amino acids that are critical to immune function. Methionine, for example, can reduce histamine levels in the body which will decrease your allergic responses and glutamine, another amino acid, is necessary for the growth of immune cells. Remember that your protein does not always have to come from animal sources like fish, eggs, and poultry. You can also obtain sufficient protein from a variety of plants such as grains, legumes, beans, nuts, and seeds.

I try and ensure, on a daily basis, that my body is getting ample amounts of all the nutrients in the above list. I want to give my immune system every advantage so it can serve me well. The above nutrients arc by no means the only way to enhance your immune function, but these are the ones that I believe have helped me live a robust and healthy life.

●　　●　　●

CHAPTER 14

Buyer Beware!

*Today, more than 95% of all chronic disease
is caused by food choice, toxic food ingredients,
nutritional deficiencies and lack of physical exercise*
— MIKE ADAMS

I don't think I can write a book about reclaiming your health without mentioning GMOs and their impact on your health. If you are not familiar with the acronym GMO, it stands for Genetically Modified Organisms. GMOs are novel organisms created in a laboratory using genetic modification and engineering techniques. In my mind, if it has been created in a laboratory it is *not* real food. It is a manufactured *food-like* product. I classify GMOs as toxic and I don't think our bodies know what to do with genetically engineered products. I am not alone in my distrust and disdain of GMOs, there are numerous scientists and consumer and environmental groups who have cited numerous health and environmental risks associated with foods containing GMOs.

Like many things, GMOs have infiltrated our daily lives without us even knowing it. There are many studies that confirm the safety of consuming GMOs and that they do *not* pose a risk to our health. The only problem I have with this is that the people doing the studies are the ones who are producing the GMOs and stand to profit from their ongoing use. How can this research be trustworthy? The following is a list of the most commonly genetically modified foods:

- Tomatoes
- Papaya (Hawaiian)
- Corn
- Soy
- Rice
- Beets
- Canola
- Squash
- Cotton (cottonseed oil)
- Potatoes

There are numerous multi-national corporations who are investing billions of dollars in the fight against the labelling of genetically modified ingredients. They clearly don't want consumers to know if their products contain GMOs. If these companies were concerned about our health and welfare, would they not want to provide us all the information we require to make an informed choice? Their concern is profit. And I believe they don't want to label their products GMO because they know it would hurt sales. They continue to assert that GMOs are not harmful to our health. But if that's the case, then why not let us know? It's up to each of us to question this and realize it's our responsibility to educate ourselves on what is in the best interests of our health instead of letting other people decide for us.

These massive corporations advertise and disseminate information about everything they are doing that is in our best interests such as offering us innovative and healthy choices, smart labelling, and keeping the industry 'green,' but the bottom line is that they are driven by profits, not the state of our health. Their information is going to be one-sided and it's going to favor their products. Personally, I don't believe a word of marketing about the processed and refined food industry. They can tell me their latest chemically-laden artificial sweetener is 'derived from nature,' but it won't sway me at the grocery store. Buyer beware! I boycott these food manufacturing companies as much as possible as I do not want to contribute to their profits. This is one way I can exercise my power and make a choice that I know is in my best long-term interests.

While there are food manufacturers selling us fake food that has the potential to make us sick, I believe the pharmaceutical industry is committed to keeping us sick. Illness and disease is a multi-billion-dollar industry and our unwellness is making a lot of people very wealthy. In the movie "What the Health" by filmmaker Kip Anderson, Kip reveals that chronic disease treatment (ie: cancer, heart disease, diabetes, etc.) is a $1.5 trillion dollar/year business in the US alone. That's the GDP equivalent of the 10th richest country in the world. That's a lot of money by any standard.

With business so good why would the pharmaceutical industry want to see an end to that kind of profit? I believe they are quite content to perpetuate illness so we continue to need their drugs. Who do you think determines whether a pharmaceutical is good for a particular symptom or ailment? It's the same company that makes that pharmaceutical; the same process used by the people manufacturing GMOs. How does this make sense? The company that makes a product should not be the one who is also testing if it's effective or safe for long-term use. That's like asking the fox to guard the hen house. The pharmaceutical industry also contributes large amounts of money to the grocery manufacturers and the various health associations so, don't expect to find the truth in any of the advertising, propaganda or literature produced by these organizations.

The pharmaceutical industry is now taking their products to the masses through TV advertising and touting how their drugs can help you live a full and symptom free life and we are getting sucked in to this way of thinking. Somehow, we have been brainwashed to believe we *need* these things to be healthy. This relates back to how our thoughts eventually become beliefs. Pharmaceuticals are chemicals that disrupt the natural chemistry of our body. They do not build us up and they do not help us address the root cause of our sickness; they just treat a symptom.

At the height of my illness, I was taking over 30 pills per day: steroids, antibiotics, antacids, immune suppressing drugs and anti-inflammatories. Not one of these pharmaceuticals were helping to resolve the underlying root cause of my illness. They were just designed to address a single symptom and, sometimes, they couldn't even control the symptom they were designed to treat. And they all had side effects. Several of the drugs I was taking were to counteract the side effects of the primary drugs. How ludicrous is that? And what was it doing to my toxic load? It was a vicious cycle, and yet all the medical professionals in my life continued to assert that these drugs were necessary to keep me healthy! Not one doctor ever suggested I could do something differently.

Perhaps you are thinking I sound a bit radical. Being sick changes you. I was so unwell for such a long time that I have now become fiercely protective of my health! It is beyond frustrating to me that we continue to be bombarded and regularly exposed to things that perpetuate illness. I feel called to stand up for what I know to be true and I know that GMOs and pharmaceuticals are not the pathway to health and vitality. I encourage you to do your own research and draw your own conclusions. Remember, knowledge is power.

• • •

CHAPTER 15

Stress Less From the Inside Out

Those who think they have no time for healthy eating,
will sooner or later have to find time for illness
— EDWARD STANLEY

I n addition to promoting physical wellness, diet and nutrition can also be powerful tools in managing mental health. We are hardwired to turn to food to feel better but, our bodies actually respond to different foods in different ways. Processed and refined junk food are actually mood busters. They may provide us short term gratification but, in the long run, they deplete us and our ability to successfully manage stress.

All emotions, thoughts, and sensory perceptions are transmitted through our nerves. Nerves are considered the electrical circuit of the body. If the circuit is overcharged due to stress, this will have a negative impact on all our body systems. Part of our nervous system is the HPA axis (hypothalamus, pituitary, and adrenals). This axis controls how we react to stress and it also regulates numerous other body processes such as digestion, mood, emotions, sexuality, and energy. It is the mechanism for interactions between glands and hormones. And, just like all other body parts, the functioning of our HPA axis is dependent on certain nutrients. Louise Hay also said if you are struggling to think positive thoughts, despite all your best efforts, look at your diet and see whether it is helping or hindering your ability to be successful. Our brain plays a large role in regulating the HPA axis and, we know that fats are vital for optimal brain function. Brain fat is made up of saturated and monounsaturated fat, cholesterol, Omega 3's (EPA and DHA) and Omega 6's (GLA and AA). The body makes the first 3 but the Omega's must come from diet. Omega 3 fats are typically the most deficient in the body (we usually get too much Omega 6 from our standard North American diet) yet, they are so important. They regulate the release and performance of neurotransmitters like dopamine, serotonin and norephinephrine – these neurotransmitters are linked to mood, anxiety, attention, alertness, energy and motivation. If you are following a low-fat diet, or getting your fat from processed food, you are most definitely deficient in Omega 3 fats and this could be having a negative impact on your ability to manage your day to day stress.

Proteins and their constituents, amino acids, comprise the communication system of the brain. Think of neurotransmitters as messengers and the words they use are made up of amino acids. As such, protein deficiency can be linked to poor communication in the brain resulting in all kinds of mental health symptoms including slow response time, reduced concentration, poor memory and even depression.

Clean, complex carbohydrates are also needed to fuel the brain. Your brain consumes more glucose than any other organ. Up to 40% of all the carbohydrates you eat are devoted to brain fuel. BUT, as we know, not all carbs are created equal. The brain craves complex whole carbohydrates for optimal function. Refined, processed and simple carbohydrates create a spike in blood sugar, insulin and adrenaline = sad brain.

Another interesting fact is that more than 90% of our serotonin receptors live in our gut. Serotonin is one of our "feel good" neurotransmitters. If more than 90% of our serotonin receptors live in our gut, then it stands to reason, an unhealthy gut can also lead to low mood, anxiety, stress, and irritability. This is another incentive to ensure you are keeping the health of your gut a top priority. Countries with higher sugar consumption have higher rates of depression; another indicator that excess sugar is damaging to the body. Other factors that can contribute to mental health issues are lack of sleep, thyroid dysfunction, adrenal fatigue, hormonal imbalance, candida, liver toxicity, underactive stomach, and excessive exposure to electromagnetic transmissions. Most pharmaceuticals create vitamin and mineral deficiencies in the body so, if you are taking any kind of drug make it your mission to know what nutrients it is depleting and whether this could be contributing to poor mental health and an inability to manage stress in your life.

The good news is that a whole foods diet can help you improve your mood, reduce anxiety and manage your stress effectively. In fact, there are foods that can deliver specific nutrients to the body allowing the brain to produce neurotransmitters that can help you feel better and enhance your emotional well being. For example, magnesium and manganese provide energy to the brain. Zinc is considered neuro-protective. Potassium, calcium and sodium aid in the transmission of brain messages. Iron carries oxygen to the brain and assists in the formation of neurotransmitters. B vitamins help protect the nervous system, enhance memory and sharpen the senses while Vitamin C protects the brain from free radical damage. In fact, Vitamin C levels are super high in the brain - 15x higher than anywhere else in the body. You can actually fight depression, and other mental health diagnoses, with nutrition!

Deficiencies in the following nutrients have all been linked to mental health issues:

- B1 — poor concentration
- B2 — depression

- B3 — depression, stress
- B5 — poor memory
- B6 — depression, poor memory, irritability, stress
- B12 — poor memory, confusion
- Folic acid — anxiety, depression
- Magnesium — anxiety, depression, irritability, stress, insomnia
- Vitamin C — depression
- Selenium — depression, irritability
- Zinc — depression, confusion, loss of appetite, lack of motivation, decreased cognitive function
- Iron — anxiety, depression
- Omega 3s — depression, anxiety, poor memory
- Tryptophan — depression
- Vitamin D — depression
- Chromium — depression
- Tyrosine — depression

By focusing on a diet rich in the above nutrients, you may be able to reduce some of your mental health symptoms and enhance your body's ability to manage stress naturally. The following is a list of foods that are abundant in these nutrients. You can use it a shopping list or as incentive to plan your meals:

- Brown rice — B1, B2, B3, B5, B6, selenium
- Asparagus — folic acid, Vitamin C
- Oatmeal porridge — B1, B3, B5, B6, selenium, chromium
- Walnuts — magnesium, Omega 3's, tryptophan, zinc
- Brazil Nuts — selenium
- Pecans — vitamin A
- Almonds — B vitamins, vitamin E
- Chia seeds — Omega 3's, iron

- Pumpkin Seeds — magnesium, zinc, Omega 3s, tyrosine
- Sunflower Seeds — magnesium, Omega 3s, zinc, selenium, vitamin E
- Hemp hearts — magnesium, zinc, Omega 3s
- Raw cacao — magnesium, zinc, iron
- Garlic — selenium, chromium
- Kidney beans — tryptophan, iron
- Avocado — B6, folic acid, essential fatty acids
- Leafy greens — magnesium, B vitamins, Vitamin C
- Peppers — B1, B3, B5, B6, Vitamin C, magnesium
- Broccoli — B1, B3, B5, B6, magnesium, chromium, selenium
- Spinach — folic acid, vitamin E, magnesium, iron
- Bananas — B6, tryptophan
- Strawberries — vitamin C
- Eggs — zinc, B2, B12, vitamin A & E
- Chicken — B12, tryptophan, tyrosine, iron
- Salmon — B12, omega 3's, selenium, zinc, tyrosine

Other nutrients that can support your mood include: probiotics, tulsi (also known as holy basil), and mushrooms such as, reishi, chaga, and lion's mane. Dried mushroom supplements are readily available everywhere these days and can be used in a variety of ways such as, in the mushroom elixir I mentioned in Gut Health 101 or throwing them in a smoothie. By now I hope we are well aware of how to get a therapeutic dose of probiotics and, if you are wondering about tulsi, it is accessible in a variety of supplements or yummy teas. Tulsi actually has a wonderful flavor when brewed in tea; it's a mild, earthy, herbal taste that is hard to resist.

• • •

CHAPTER 16

The Skinny on Fat

*Don't eat anything your great great
grandmother wouldn't recognize as food*
— MICHAEL POLLAN

I think it's safe to say we have been duped about fat. Everything we have ever been told about fat, and fat consumption, is wrong. Fat does amazing things for the body. I have already explained the benefits of good fat but, for the record, let's review it one more time. Good fat helps stabilize blood sugar levels and it ensures we can absorb and utilize fat soluble vitamins such as, A, D, and E. Good fat is very neuro-protective and is critical to keep our brain functioning at optimal levels. Good fat helps manage appetite and decrease intense food cravings. Good fat supports our immune system, makes our skin soft and supple and keeps us healthy. Good fat does *not* make you fat and *good* fat does not raise cholesterol levels. But, unfortunately, fat has a bad reputation and I would like to try and set the record straight.

Cholesterol has been demonized by traditional western medicine. Cholesterol is in every cell of the body; it helps conduct nerve impulses, it helps produce bile for digestion and detoxification, it is involved in the production of stress and sex hormones, it helps to waterproof the skin, it supports the production of vitamin D in the body, it protects against depression and aging, and it helps us fight off cancer. It makes up 20% of brain tissue. It's so important the body manufactures about 80% of the cholesterol we require. The other 20% comes from diet. But cholesterol is so important to our bodies that if we decrease the amount of fat we are eating the body just ends up manufacturing *more*. In fact, if you are vegan, the body will produce 100% of what you need. To be clear, cholesterol is *vital* to our health.

The ongoing belief that cholesterol is bad for the body dates back to a study in 1952. That's over 50 years old and, in today's world, research and information that's over 5 years old is outdated. In 1952, Mr. Ancel Keys published a report showing a *supposed* correlation between the consumption of fats and cholesterol and the incidence of heart disease in six countries. Unfortunately, the study was biased. Mr. Keys had data from 22 countries, including France and Polynesia, where they consume *high* fat diets with little to no heart disease, but because this data did *not* support his hypothesis he excluded it and chose only the six countries that supported his preconceived notion. If he had included all the data there would have be no correlation between fat consumption and increased risk of heart disease. In fact, more up to date research demonstrates that as many as 50–80% of people who have heart attacks do not have elevated levels of cholesterol (The Cholesterol Myths, Uffe Ravnskov, MD, PhD and The Nutritional Bypass David W. Rowland).

For optimal health, the goal is to decrease the HDL (the bad fat) and increase the LDL (the good, healthy, protective fat). This is not necessarily done by avoiding fat. Interestingly enough, current research is now showing that while bad fats and trans fat will increase cholesterol serum levels, it's sugar, alcohol, caffeine, and smoking that have the biggest impact on our bad cholesterol levels. Good dietary fat from avocado, eggs, butter, nuts, seeds, olive oil, flax, and coconut oil will actually decrease the bad cholesterol and increase the good. Other things that will improve the good LDL include fiber, supplementing with probiotics, vitamin B, anti-oxidants, exercise, and avoiding inflammatory foods. We have also been told to avoid ALL saturated fats because they raise our risk of cardiovascular disease. We now know this is patently false (if it was true, our rates of cardiovascular disease should be declining and yet they continue to rise). Coconut oil has recently been vilified again with claims that it is a saturated fat and should not be consumed freely. Coconut oil is different from other saturated fats, it's a medium chain triglyceride meaning the body can use it readily for energy compared to long chain triglycerides which the body stores as fat. Coconut oil is also stable at high heat, this means you can cook with it and it does not oxidize and become rancid or carcinogenic. Coconut oil is also anti-fungal, anti-bacterial, and anti-microbial. Organic butter, another saturated fat, is full of vital minerals and vitamins and, as stated earlier, it contains butyric acid, a short chain triglyceride which the body loves to use to restore the lining of the gut. Butyric acid is also anti-fungal, anti-bacterial, and anti-microbial. And, like coconut oil, it's stable at high heat and can also be used for cooking. I use both of these fats in my kitchen and have no intention of limiting their consumption.

And what about poly & mono unsaturated fats? Polyunsaturated fats and oils have many health benefits; however, they are highly unstable. They will oxidize when exposed to heat, light, and air. Once these oils have oxidized, they become a source of free radicals and, when ingested, we know that free radicals wreak havoc in the body damaging healthy cells. This means you should *never* cook with your polyunsaturated oils such as olive, flax, or grapeseed oils as they go rancid when heated. You should also purchase these oils in dark colored glass bottles to reduce their exposure to light. And, to protect them against overexposure to air, buy them in smaller bottles as this helps ensure the oil stays fresh. If you are buying the big family sized jug, your oil has gone rancid by the time you are halfway through that bottle. So, polyunsaturated fats are great for salad dressings, homemade mayonnaise, and anything else that does not involve heat. A discussion on fat would not be complete without mentioning Omega 3 fats. Omega 3s regulate the release and performance of neurotransmitters like dopamine, serotonin, and norepinephrine — as we know, these neurotransmitters are linked to mood, anxiety, attention, alertness, energy and motivation. Two very important sources of Omega 3 fats are EPA and DHA. These particular fats can be obtained from cold water fish such as salmon, black cod, halibut, and sardines. We can also obtain EPA and DHA from avocado oil, macadamia nut oil, walnuts, and pecans. The health benefits of EPA and DHA cannot be overstated. They reduce inflammation, support the nervous system, enhance brain function, improve nerve transmission, aid weight loss, boost immunity, improve skin health, reduce PMS... the list goes on. If you are not supplementing with EPA or DHA consider adding it to your regimen as it is difficult to obtain an optimal level of these through diet alone.

As outlined in earlier chapters, there are bad fats that are actually damaging to our body, these are the trans fats and hydrogenated fats, and they are implicated in numerous serious health conditions. Trans and hydrogenated fats are free radicals and once ingested, they promote inflammation, interfere with basic cell membrane function, displace good fat, and wreak havoc anywhere and everywhere. This damage can pave the way for cancer, diabetes, neurological conditions (trans fats have an affinity for brain tissue), and cardiovascular conditions. Trans fats and hydrogenated oils are in the vast majority of processed foods, including various kinds of chips, margarine, cake mixes and frostings, pancake and waffle mixes, nondairy creamers, microwave popcorn, packaged cookies, blended creamy drinks, many packaged crackers, prepared puddings, and fried foods. It's so important to understand the differences between good and bad fat so you can make better choices.

The bottom line is, don't be afraid of fat! Good, healthy dietary fat does a body good. Remember: quality is important. Toxins and chemicals tend to concentrate in fats, so choosing organic will reduce your toxic load. Cook with coconut oil and organic butter, use polyunsaturated oils (olive, flax) in your salad dressings, throw in a good dose of omega 3s, and remember to supplement with fish oil. Your body will thank you.

● ● ●

Part IV — Life After Crohn's

CHAPTER 17
Blessings

Take care of your body. It's the only
place you have to live
— JIM ROHN

I t's been over 25 years since I was originally diagnosed with Crohn's disease. In the early years, I often wondered why I got Crohn's. I understand now that it was part of my journey and recovering from Crohn's helped me find my true passion in life — holistic nutrition!! And I want to share my passion with everyone and anyone who will listen.

I believe whole heartedly that the "5 Steps to Total Wellness" saved my life. And not only saved my life, but have allowed me to thrive over the last 20 years. Supposedly, because of my Crohn's diagnosis I am considered vulnerable (like babies and frail old people), but I am far from vulnerable. I experience a level of health that most people can't imagine! When I was sick, it felt like the disease dictated every aspect of my life. In some respects, I felt like a prisoner. Once I started to actually nourish my body and reclaimed my health, a whole new world opened up to me.

Over the last 17 years, I have been able to engage in activities I had only dreamed about previously. My husband and I have travelled extensively — Costa Rica, Vietnam, Mexico, London, Paris, New York, San Francisco, and San Diego to name a few of the places we have visited. I volunteered in India, Burma, and Thailand with a group called Medical Mercy, for three months back in 2006 and I didn't have to worry about my health. I was eating local food, being exposed to all kinds of new bugs and bacteria, and travelling in remote and isolated locations including the jungle and countryside, and yet I was able to stay healthy. Many other volunteers became sick with dysentery and traveler's diarrhea, but I maintained a level of physical strength the entire trip! I also became a Certified Fitness Instructor once I became well. I taught a variety of classes including aerobics and strength training for many years. Once again, this was not anything I could have dreamed of doing when I was sick. In 2009, I also participated in a triathlon just because I could. All of these accomplishments and milestones remind me how blessed I am to have found my way back to my own power and to have reclaimed my health in ways I didn't know possible.

Presently, I continue to enjoy excellent health and I spend my time consulting with clients on how to reclaim their own health. I host Louise Hay workshops periodically because I believe that good mental and emotional health are paramount to overall well-being. I produce a podcast series called Healthy Ever After and I post health related videos on YouTube for anyone who is interested in feeling better. I still workout regularly because moving your body is a critical component to staying fit, vital, and in living a long life.

I have five grandchildren whom I enjoy spending time with and I still have the energy to do lots of fun things with them. I have a wonderful and fabulous marriage that is fulfilling and rewarding. I *love* walking my dog and spending time with him — he teaches me about living in the moment. I meditate every day and participate in my daily devotion practice where I give thanks for all the things that are going well in my life; and there are numerous things going well. Several years ago, my husband and I were able to purchase a second home in Carlsbad, California, and we travel there often to spend time at the beach and get some sun and humidity. It's always a welcome relief from the dryness of where I live. I feel incredibly thankful to be enjoying life and I know that if I had not made the dietary changes I made back in 2001, I would not be where I am today. There is no doubt in my mind that those changes paved the way for the wonderful life I now live.

I continue to be astounded at how my body works. It speaks to me daily and informs me what it needs and what it dislikes. As long as I stay in tune with my body and listen to all the ways it communicates, I am able to maintain optimal health. I have complete and total faith in my innate ability to be well. Now I have intentions of living in to my 90s and 100s with robust health. I am not the least bit interested in being sick and I know that if I take care of my body, it will provide me with everything I need to continue living for many years to come!

I am deeply grateful for the time you took to read my story. My hope is that the information has inspired you, in some way, to rethink your approach to health. I know from firsthand experience that we do have the ability to reclaim our wellness. I believe, 110%, that the body knows what to do if we give it the tools it needs. We do not have to live lives full of illness, pain, disability, and death! Our bodies are not designed for sickness; they are designed for robust, vibrant, health and I encourage you to reclaim what you have lost through some basic diet and lifestyle changes. My most sincere wish for all of you is to live "healthy ever after".

● ● ●

APPENDIX

6£

MISERICORDIA HOSPITAL
16940 - 87 AVENUE
EDMONTON, ALBERTA
T5R 4H5
(403) 484-8811

LIMA, Patti   555773

Dr. D. Adams

REPORT OF OPERATION:

DATE: May 6/91   ANESTHETIST: Dr. E. Chan
SURGEON: Dr. D. Adams   ASSISTANT(S): Dr. Daudi   Dr. Connick
ANESTHESIA START: 1140   SURGERY START: 1150   SURGERY END: 1325

PREOPERATIVE DIAGNOSIS: CROHN DISEASE

PROPOSED OPERATION: SEGMENTAL RESECTION OF MIDTRANSVERSE COLON PLUS
                          RIGHT HEMICOLECTOMY FOR A STENOTIC SEGMENT AT THE
                          TERMINAL ILEUM NEAR THE ILEOCECAL VALVE

OPERATION PERFORMED: SAME

POSTOPERATIVE DIAGNOSIS: SAME

INDICATIONS: This is a 25-year-old married woman who presented with increasing
symptoms of diarrhea, abdominal pain and cramps. She had had these symptoms for
5 years but a diagnosis of Crohn was only made a year and a half ago. She had
been treated medically with high dose steroids. However, in spite of this
medical regimen, she had had a fixed stenotic segment in the midtransverse colon
and terminal ileum near the ileocecal valve. Because of this pathology that was
refractory to medical treatment, she was considered for elective resection.

FINDINGS: Normal small bowel up to a stenotic segment just proximal to the
ileocecal valve. Another stenotic segment in the midtransverse colon. Just
proximal to our ileocecal anastomosis, about 30-35 cm from the ileocecal valve,
there were two additional areas of creeping fat and slight thickening of the
bowel. Because this was considered to be mild involvement, these segments were
left alone. After the anastomosis was completed, they were 10 cm proximal to
the ileocolic anastomosis.

PROCEDURE: Once general anesthesia was administered, the patient was prepped
and draped in the usual fashion. Through a transverse incision that was
slightly slanted superiorly at the midline, entry was gained into the peritoneal
cavity. Electrocautery was used to control bleeders. Electrocautery was used
to divide the anterior rectus sheath and the rectus muscle. The posterior
rectus sheath and peritoneum were grasped between two hemostats and divided
sharply. This incision was extended in either direction with the Metzenbaum
scissors and the electrocautery. Once into the peritoneal cavity, the findings
mentioned above were evident. The cecum was mobilized by dividing along the
avascular white line of Toldt. The lateral peritoneal attachments to the cecum
were thus freed and dissection both superiorly and inferiorly allowed us to

continued page 2

DATE   PHYSICIAN'S SIGNATURE

135

MISERICORDIA HOSPITAL
16940 - 87 AVENUE
EDMONTON, ALBERTA
T5R 4H5
(403) 484-8811

LIMA, Patti   555773

Dr. D. Adams

REPORT OF OPERATION:

Page 2

deliver the cecum and ileum into the incision. The areas of disease were
outlined. Our resection margins were mapped out. The proximal resection margin
was to include 30 cm of terminal ileum and approx 10 cm of cecum in continuity.
The mesentery between these two points were scored and then controlled with
hemostats and 2-0 Dexon ties. The bowel was divided with cutting current on the
electrocautery. We then performed our ileocolic anastomosis. The anastomosis
was performed with 4-0 silk in single layer interrupted fashion. Once the
anastomosis was completed, patency and integrity of the anastomosis was
verified. The mesenteric defect was sewn up with 3-0 Dexon in a running
fashion.
      Next, our attention turned to the midtransverse colon lesion. The
gastrocolic ligament was dissected free of the colon and the mesentery was
skeletonized. Then, we decided upon our resection margins. This was to be a
very conservative resection with approx a 1-2 cm clearance on either side of the
fixed lesion. The mesentery was scored, controlled with hemostats and 2-0 Dexon
ties. The segment of bowel was excised with cutting current on the
electrocautery. Next, we performed our colocolonic anastomosis. This was again
performed with 4-0 silk in single layer simple interrupted fashion. The
integrity and patency of the anastomosis was verified. Mesenteric defect was
sutured up with 3-0 Dexon in a running fashion. A final check was made for
hemostasis. We irrigated the peritoneal cavity with saline. Satisfied with our
hemostasis, our attention turned towards closure. Closure was accomplished by
running #1 Dexon in posterior rectus sheath and anterior rectus sheath. Skin
was closed with vertical mattress interrupted 3-0 Surgilene sutures and
intervening skin segments were Steri-Stripped. No drains were used. The
patient tolerated the procedure well and there were no complications. Sponge,
needle and instrument counts were correct on two separate occasions. This was
verified by manual and visual inspection of the operative site. Blood loss was
less than 200 ml. The patient left for Recovery in satisfactory condition.

D. May 6/91
T. May 7/91

cc: Dr. D. Adams
    Dr. M. Millan
    Dr. Daudi (Resident)

Dr. Daudi dictating
Dr. D. Adams/jv

DATE   PHYSICIAN'S SIGNATURE

S1290 /1870A31

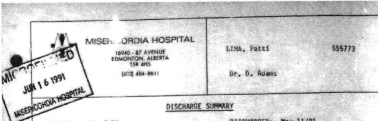

MISERICORDIA HOSPITAL
16940 - 87 AVENUE
EDMONTON, ALBERTA
T5R 4H5
(403) 484-8811

LIMA, Patti   555773

Dr. D. Adams

DISCHARGE SUMMARY

ADMITTED: May 5/91   DISCHARGED: May 11/91

COMPLAINTS AND DURATION: This 25-year-old female was admitted for resection of
her Crohn disease. She had been known to have Crohn disease for one and half
years, however probably had had symptoms for five years. She had been well
until December of 1990 when she had had a very severe flare-up. Recent
colonoscopy demonstrated that she had segmental involvement of the mid-portion
of her transverse colon and also had marked stenosis of her terminal ileum. Dr.
Millan had felt that she was now a candidate for surgery. She was having
increasing amounts of abdominal cramping and bloating. She was also
experiencing increasing diarrhea.
    Present medications included prednisone 25 mg daily, and she was also on
Imuran, iron, and the birth control pill.
PAST HISTORY: Included ████████████████████████, and tonsillectomy five
years previously. She had been hospitalized and treated conservatively in July
of 1990 for a bowel obstruction secondary to her Crohn disease.
FUNCTIONAL INQUIRY: Essentially normal.
PHYSICAL EXAMINATION: She was a healthy 25-year-old female. Blood pressure
110/70, pulse 76. Head and neck - nothing abnormal detected. Chest clear.
Cardiovascular system normal. Examination of the abdomen demonstrated some
tenderness in the right lower quadrant. The remainder of her examination was
essentially within normal limits. ██████████████████████████████████████.
LABORATORY WORK-UP ON ADMISSION: SMA-12 normal. Electrolytes normal.
Urinalysis clear. Hemoglobin 14.4 grams, white count 11,600. Blood grouping
was O+.
PROGRESS IN HOSPITAL: On the 6th of May, a right hemicolectomy and segmental
resection of the mid-transverse colon was performed. Pathology report
demonstrated Crohn disease of the terminal ileum and also Crohn disease of the
transverse colon, both of which appeared to be quite active. Her postoperative
course was excellent. Her diet was advanced rapidly. She was discharged home
on a full diet on the 11th of May with prescriptions for oral analgesics and
plans to decrease her prednisone over the following four weeks. She will be
reviewed in the office in two weeks.

D: May 22/91
T: May 27/91
cc: Dr. D. Adams , Dr. M. Millan

MOST RESPONSIBLE DIAGNOSIS: CROHN DISEASE OF TERMINAL ILEUM AND MID-TRANSVERSE
                               COLON.

Dr. D. Adams/mpTypeMed   3/Jun/91   X
                              DATE   PHYSICIAN'S SIGNATURE

MISERICORDIA HOSPITAL
16940 - 87 AVENUE
EDMONTON, ALBERTA
T5R 4H5
(403) 484-8811

LIMA, Patti   555773

Dr. D. Adams

DISCHARGE SUMMARY

ADMISSION DATE: May 16, 1991   DISCHARGE DATE: May 21, 1991

CLINICAL HISTORY: This 25-year-old female was readmitted through the emergency
department ...th of May 1991 with severe abdominal pain. She had undergone
... ...ections for Crohn's on May 6, 1991, and had an excellent
... ...til the day of admission when she suddenly developed severe
... ...ain. She had had no nausea or vomiting and bowels had been
... ...happened. She was presently on prednisone 15 mg daily and

... strated that she has had one bowel resection. She also had

... ...ry was essentially negative.

PHYSICAL EXAMINATION: She was a distressed 25-year-old female with obvious
abdominal pain. One was afebrile. Blood pressure 120/73. Pulse 100. Head and
neck ...g abnormal detected. Chest clear. Cardiovascular system: Heart
sounds normal. Examination of the abdomen demonstrated a quite rigid abdomen in
the right side. Bowel sounds were present but decreased. The right lower
quadrant incision was healing well. Liver, spleen, and both kidneys were neither
palpable nor tender. Hernial sites were clear. Rectal examination was
unimpressive. The remainder of her examination was essentially within normal
limits.

LABORATORY DATA: On admission SMA-12: Alkaline phosphatase 116, urea 7.2.
Electrolytes were basically normal, except for a slightly low potassium which was
corrected. Amylase was normal. Urinalysis was clear. Pregnancy test was
negative. Hemoglobin 14.7 g, white count 19.50 with a shift to the left. Blood
cultures showed no growth. A urinary culture was inclusive. Cervical swab showed
no pathology.

X-RAY FINDINGS: Previews of the abdomen were nonspecific, and when repeated
showed a slightly dilated small bowel. Ultrasound of the abdomen demonstrated a
very small capsular perirenal amount of fluid.

TREATMENT AND PROGRESS: Believing that she had a small leak from her anastomosis,
which was localized, she was admitted, given analgesics, and placed on intravenous
crystalloid and was administered Cefoxitin 2 g every six hours. She was also
covered with Solu-Cortef. In the following three days she became markedly better.
She remained basically afebrile. She was followed by Dr. Millan. By the 18th she
was on fluids and on the 19th was placed back on prednisone and off Solu-Cortef.

DISCHARGE MANAGEMENT PLAN: She was discharged home on the 21st, eating a full
diet and feeling much better.

OPERATION:

CONSULTANTS:

D. May 27, 1991
T. May 31, 1991

Continued page 2...

DATE   PHYSICIAN'S SIGNATURE

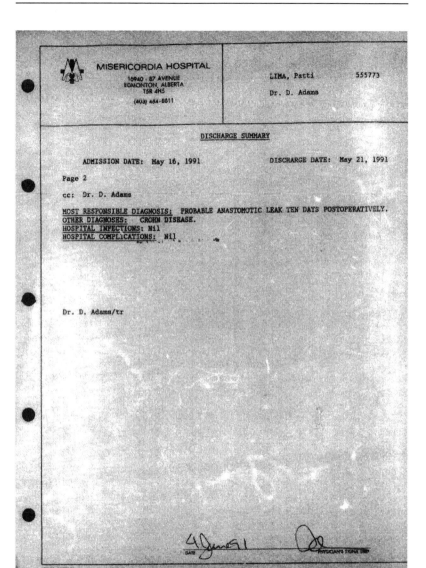

MISERICORDIA HOSPITAL
16940 - 87 AVENUE
EDMONTON, ALBERTA
T5R 4H5
(403) 484-8011

LIMA, Patti   555773

Dr. D. Adams

DISCHARGE SUMMARY

ADMISSION DATE: May 16, 1991   DISCHARGE DATE: May 21, 1991

Page 2

cc: Dr. D. Adams

MOST RESPONSIBLE DIAGNOSIS: PROBABLE ANASTOMOTIC LEAK TEN DAYS POSTOPERATIVELY.
OTHER DIAGNOSES: CROHN DISEASE.
HOSPITAL INFECTIONS: Nil
HOSPITAL COMPLICATIONS: Nil

Dr. D. Adams/tr

Manufactured by Amazon.ca
Bolton, ON